THE COMPLETE GUIDE TO

Anita Bean

STRENGTH TRAINING

3rd edition

A & C Black • London

Published in 2005 by A & C Black Publishers Ltd
37 Soho Square, London W1D 3QZ
www.acblack.com

Third Edition 2005
First Edition 1997; reprinted 1998, 1999 and 2000; Second Edition 2001

ISBN 0 7136 6040 6

A CIP catalogue record for this book is available from the British Library.

Acknowledgements
Cover photograph courtesy of Corbis.
Photography by Grant Pritchard.
Illustrations by James Wakelin.

Typeset in 10½ on 12pt Palatino

Printed and bound in Singapore by Tien Wah Press Pte.

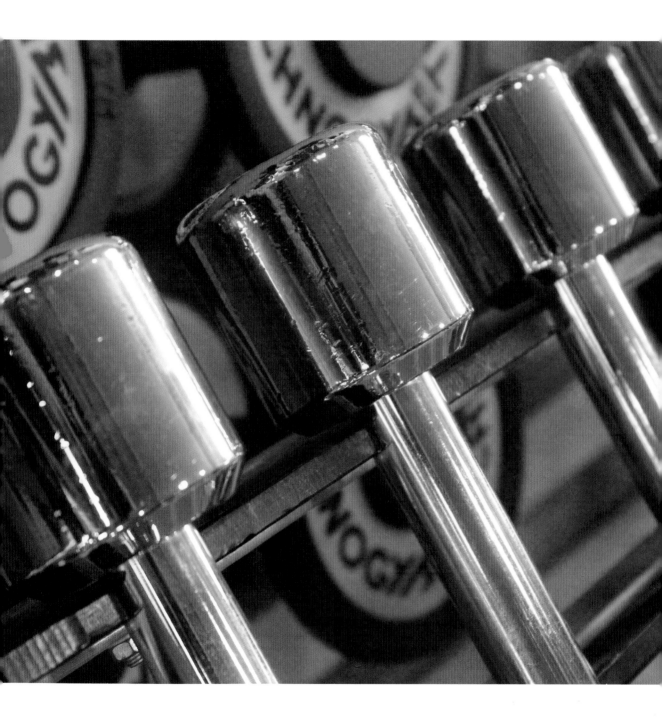

CONTENTS

LIST OF ABBREVIATIONS

1RM	One-rep max		GH	Growth hormone
ATP	Adenosine Triphosphate		HR	Heart rate
bpm	Beats per minute		IAAs	Indispensable amino acids
BV	Biological value		MHR	Maximum heart rate
BCAAs	Branched chained amino acids		MRP	Meal replacement product
DAAs	Dispensable amino acids		ORAC	Oxygen Radical Absorbance Capacity
DHA	Docosahexanoic acid		PC	Phosphocreatine
DPA	Docosapentanoic acid		ROM	Range of movement
EPA	Eicosapentanoic acid		RPE	Rating of perceived exertion
EPOC	Excess post-exercise oxygen consumption		RDA	Recommended daily amount
			Reps	Repetitions
FT	Fast twitch		RMR	Resting metabolic rate
GLA	Gamma-linolenic acid		ST	Slow twitch
GI	Glycaemic index		THR	Training heart rate
GTOs	Golgi tendon organs			

FOREWORD BY BOB SMITH

I first met Anita many years ago when we lectured on the YMCA's fitness training courses. I noticed then how she was very interested in the education behind fitness and nutrition. Today this book represents the fulfilment of that interest and I was delighted when asked to write the Foreword, not only because I know Anita, but because the third edition of *The Complete Guide to Strength Training* is written with considerable expertise and I am certain it will go a long way to helping people achieve their goals.

Strength training is probably the most eclectic form of fitness training, meaning that many techniques and systems work for a variety of different people. No one approach is necessarily better than another, but a full understanding of a number of approaches is very helpful. A book about strength training therefore needs to be both comprehensive and varied. It requires a large number of ideas and strategies to cater for individual requirements, goals, body types and personalities.

Anita has successfully combined all of these ingredients, resulting in a book that is comprehensive, accurate and written in an easy to follow style. Additional information is provided about surrounding issues such as diet, fat loss and muscle physiology, which is both helpful and necessary. In *The Complete Guide to Strength Training* the reader will discover an invaluable resource suitable for any professional involved in fitness training as well as the individual wishing to gain more from their time at the gym.

Enjoy!

Bob Smith M.A. (dist) B.Ed (Hons); Cert Ed (dist);
Senior Strength and Conditioning Coach
English Institute of Sport

ACKNOWLEDGEMENTS

To my husband, Simon, for his unfailing support, and to my daughters, Chloe and Lucy for providing my inspiration.

Many thanks to Grant Pritchard for the great photography (and making everyone laugh) and to personal trainer Steve Tunstall for demonstrating the exercises with such proficiency.

I am grateful to past editor Penny Clarke for her vision, and to my current editor Claire Dunn at A & C Black for her expertise and for making this book possible.

Photos were shot on location at Holmes Place, Epsom.

PREFACE TO THE THIRD EDITION

I wrote the first edition of The Complete Guide to Strength Training in 1997 as a tribute to my success as a natural bodybuilding champion (EFBB British Lightweight Champion, 1991) and to encapsulate the fulfilment I had experienced from 15 years of strength training. I wanted to share with you my professional knowledge as a nutritionist and fitness instructor, as well as my first-hand experience as a competitor. I am passionate about training and believe everyone can benefit from it, both physically and mentally.

This book translates the current science of training and nutrition into practical advice. It provides you with an integrated plan of action to achieve your training goals. I have drawn together scientifically proven training methods and cutting-edge nutritional advice to devise training programmes for beginners, intermediates and advanced trainers.

Part One of this book unravels the science of muscle growth and exercise nutrition. Part Two provides an illustrated, step-by-step guide to the exercises included in the training programmes, with comprehensive training technique tips. Motivation and goal-setting are covered in Part Three, as well as clear explanations of training principles, training methods and programme design. All this information is consolidated in the training programmes presented in Part Four, where I have detailed week-by-week workouts for beginners, intermediates and advanced trainers.

In this third edition I have expanded and updated the information. The book has undoubtedly benefited enormously from a new design and inspiring new photographs of every exercise. I have added new exercises and training tips in Part Two. With more emphasis now on core training, I have included new strength exercises using the exercise ball and the principles of Pilates training. I have modified and extended the training programmes according to level of experience and workout goals. There are enough workouts in this edition of the book to keep you progressing for many years to come! In response to numerous requests since the last edition of the book was published, I have devised more weights workouts for different sports, including football, rugby, swimming and running.

Throughout the text I have included references to the original sources of information, giving you the opportunity to delve further into particular topics if you wish.

Although I no longer compete, I continue to train with weights three times a week. In addition, I include lots of core training, as well as stretching and cardiovascular exercise for all-round fitness. As you can probably guess, I am a great believer in balanced training, nutrition and health. It's not always easy, of course! Like most, I too have to fit my training around a busy work schedule (as well as being mum to two beautiful daughters). Over the years, though, I have at least achieved consistency and progress in my training.

I wish you every success in achieving your own training goals, and hope you benefit from the knowledge imparted in this book.

Enjoy!

Anita Bean

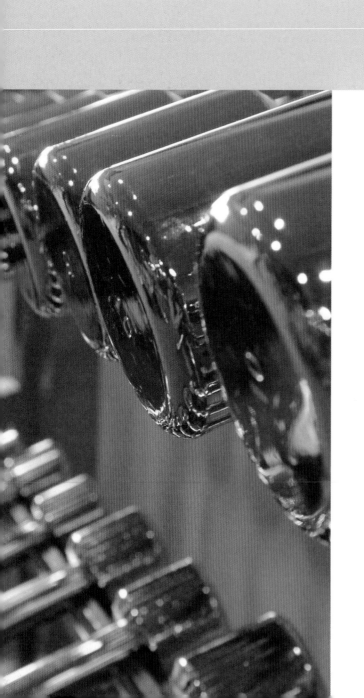

PART **ONE**

MUSCLE SCIENCE

A stronger, leaner, fitter body is within your grasp. By picking up this book, you've made a commitment to change. Whether you want to tone up, develop muscle size or improve your performance in sport, this book will help you achieve your goals. But first, a good understanding of how your muscles work, how they grow and what you need to eat will enable you to target your training more effectively. The following three chapters equip you with the training and nutritional know-how you need to get started on the road to success.

THE BENEFITS OF STRENGTH TRAINING

Strength training is not only about lifting weights and building muscle. It's also about creating a balanced musculature that can move with grace and fluidity, respond optimally to any physical demand, perform well in sport, minimise injury risk and – importantly – be aesthetically pleasing. Training with weights also develops your inner strength, gives you a terrific sense of accomplishment, builds confidence and fosters a positive mental attitude.

REASONS TO STRENGTH TRAIN

A well-planned and well-executed strength training programme can bring numerous benefits.

Increased muscle mass and strength

A well-planned weight training programme increases muscle size and strength. In contrast, endurance activities do not produce significant changes in strength or muscle mass. Research has shown that a basic weight training programme lasting just 25 minutes followed three times a week can increase muscle mass by about 1 kg over an eight-week period,[1] while lean mass gains of 20 per cent of your starting body weight are common after the first year of training.

Stronger tendons and ligaments

Weight training increases the strength of the tendons and ligaments, and therefore improves joint stability. It stimulates the production of collagen proteins in the tendons and ligaments,[1] thus causing an increase in their structural strength.

Increased metabolic rate

Strength training increases the resting metabolic rate (RMR) – the rate at which your body burns calories – by increasing muscle mass. Muscle has a higher energy requirement than fat tissue, which means the more muscle you have, the higher your metabolic rate. Research has shown that adding 1.4 kg of muscle increases RMR by 7 per cent and daily calorie requirement by 15 per cent.[2] At rest, 0.45 kg of muscle tissue requires 35 kcal/day. During exercise, energy expenditure rises dramatically – five to ten times above the resting level. Thus, the more muscle tissue you have, the greater the number of calories expended during exercise and at rest.

Anti-ageing benefits

Without exercise, adults typically experience a 2–5 per cent decrease in their metabolic rate and an increase of 7 kg of fat every decade.[3,7] This is due largely to a loss of muscle tissue and may translate into unwanted body fat gain. Without strength training, adults typically lose 2.3–3.2 kg muscle every decade.[2,3] Muscle loss occurs mainly in the fast-twitch (FT) muscle fibres, which are involved in strength and explosive activities (see pp. 8–9). This cannot be prevented by cardiovascular exercise – only strength training maintains muscle mass and strength as you get older. Therefore, strength training is an excellent way of preserving muscle mass, preventing a reduction of metabolic rate and avoiding fat gain with age.

Reduced body fat

Strength training can help reduce body fat by increasing the metabolic rate and therefore daily calorie expenditure. One study found that strength training produced a loss of 1.8 kg of fat after three months of training, despite a 15 per cent increase in calorie intake.[1] Another study of 282 adult beginners found that after eight weeks of strength training and aerobic exercise, they lost almost 4 kg fat and gained 1.4 kg muscle – a significant improvement in body composition.

Increased bone density

Strength training improves bone strength, and increases bone protein and mineral content.[4] Studies show that the bones under the most stress from weight training have the highest bone mineral content.[5] For example, it has been shown that there are significant increases in the bone mineral content of the upper femur (thigh) after four months of strength training.[6] A US study found that women who followed a weight training programme twice a week for one year developed 76 per cent more bone strength than those who did no strength training. These findings suggest, then, that weight training reduces the risk of osteoporosis and bone fractures.[6]

Reduced blood pressure

Strength training has been shown to lower both systolic and diastolic blood pressure. The effect is even greater if strength training is combined with aerobic training. An American study found that a combination of two months of strength training and aerobic exercise resulted in a decrease in systolic blood pressure of 5 mm Hg, and diastolic blood pressure of 3 mm Hg[8] (note that 'mm Hg' stands for 'mm of mercury', which is the standard unit of measurement for blood pressure).

Reduced blood cholesterol and blood fats

Studies have demonstrated improvements in blood cholesterol and blood triglycerides (fats) as a result of several weeks of strength training.[4,9]

Improved posture

Strength training greatly improves overall posture, as well as correcting specific postural faults. A number of factors influence our posture, including skeletal structure, basic body type, strength and flexibility. Obviously, the first and second factors are controlled by our genetic make-up and cannot be altered. However, strength and flexibility can be changed through training or disuse (i.e. increased or decreased demand). Imbalances in these two components lead to postural faults, but these may be corrected through specific strength training exercises and stretches.

Injury prevention

A well-conditioned and well-balanced musculoskeletal system has a much smaller chance of sustaining injury. A stronger body is better able to avoid or resist impact injuries from falls and activities such as running or jumping. Muscular imbalances are a common cause of injury: for example, underdeveloped hamstrings (back of the thighs) relative to the quadriceps (front of the thighs) can make the knee joint unstable, thus increasing injury risk.

The majority of lower-back problems are due to weakness or imbalance of the deep muscles close to the spine and pelvis, which contribute to core stability (see pp. 138–9). A well-designed strength training programme will improve the strength of the trunk stabilisers – the transverse abdominis and the lumbar multifidus – thus reducing the likelihood of injury. One study found that patients suffering lower-back pain had significantly less pain after 10 weeks of specific strength exercises.[10]

Improved psychological well-being

Consistent strength training helps to reduce stress, anxiety and depression, uplift your mood, and promote more restful sleep. It may help decrease muscle tension due to the intensity of the muscular contractions. It also improves body image, which has a major effect on psychological well-being. Participants report that they have more energy, greater confidence and that they are prouder of their appearance.

Improved appearance

Personal appearance is greatly improved by strength training due to increased muscle tone, strength, function and improved posture. Changes in body composition mean an increase in lean mass and decrease in fat mass, both of which greatly enhance the way you look.

STRENGTH TRAINING MYTHS

Despite the well-recognised benefits of strength training discussed above, there are many myths that still exist.

Myth 1: strength training makes women too bulky

Some women avoid strength training for fear that they will look too masculine. On the con-trary, strength training actually enhances a woman's femininity. It improves muscle tone and definition, and creates a better body shape. Increases in muscle mass can be made, but women can never achieve the muscle bulk of men. This is due to the fact that men have 10 times as much of the muscle-building hormone, testosterone, in their systems. Women are, there-fore, genetically programmed not to achieve the muscle bulk of men.

Myth 2: if you stop training, muscle turns to fat

It is impossible for muscle to turn to fat, as it is a completely different type of body tissue. Muscle mass and strength will gradually decrease if you stop training (some physiologists believe that a muscle will never quite return to its pre-training state), and fat stores will increase if you eat more calories than you need over a period of time. However, one will not turn into the other! Once a certain muscle mass has been achieved through regular strength training this can be maintained by training less frequently (once or twice a week).

Myth 3: strength training makes you muscle-bound and decreases flexibility

Increasing your muscle mass does not make you muscle-bound, reduce your flexibility or reduce your speed in athletic activities. On the contrary, if you train correctly – performing each exercise in strict form through a full range of motion (ROM) that gives your muscles and joints a full stretch – you can maintain and even improve flexibility. Your ROM may decrease when you lift heavy weights, so compensate for this by doing full ROM stretches between sets and espe-cially at the end of your workout.

Continued use of heavier weights, partial rep-etitions and performing exercises with an incom-plete ROM ('cheating reps') usually results in reduced flexibility. Also, if you have one muscle group (e.g. the quadriceps) that is over-developed in comparison with the opposing group (e.g. the hamstrings), this can cause reduced flexibility in that opposing muscle group. This is common in cyclists and footballers due to the larger volume of work performed by the quadriceps. In any case, stretching the relevant muscles after training will help prevent them shortening and increase their flexibility.

It has been demonstrated that a strong muscle can contract more quickly and generate more power than a weak one. In fact, the physiques of world-class sprinters are very muscular, which goes to prove that increased muscle mass does not hinder your speed or your flexibility.

Myth 4: strength training harms the joints

When performed properly and safely, strength training improves the strength of the ligaments that hold a joint together (see p. 2), thus making the joint more stable and less prone to injury. Impact movements such as running and jumping can unduly stress the ligaments and make the joints more susceptible to injury. The controlled, no-impact movements used in strength training, however, place far less stress on the joints than most other forms of exercise, and are therefore a good way of strengthening them.

THE ABC OF MUSCLE GROWTH

How do muscles get bigger? If you lift weights, eat and rest, your muscles grow. True, but the science behind it all goes much deeper. This chapter tells you how muscles are made up, how they work and how they get bigger. The more you know, the more easily you will reach your training goals.

MUSCLE FITNESS

Strength training can develop three components of muscle fitness: strength, endurance and power. The amount of weight lifted, the speed of movement and the number of repetitions will determine which aspect is developed most. In general, using heavy weights for a lower number of repetitions (fewer than 12) develops strength and size; using lighter weights for a higher number of repetitions develops endurance; explosive movements develop power.

Muscular strength

Muscular strength is the amount of force a muscle can produce – for example, the amount of weight that can be lifted. This is developed by heavy weights. Generally, the larger the muscle, the stronger it is, although other factors such as neuromuscular adaptation (the number of fibres controlled and recruited by your nervous system) affect your strength as well.

Muscular endurance

Muscular endurance is the ability of a muscle to continue contracting against a resistance. This is developed by maintaining a constant workload for increasing periods of time – lifting a weight for 12 or more repetitions then building up to, say, 15, 20 and so on, as endurance improves. Long-distance cycling will develop muscle endurance in the thigh muscles, for example.

Muscular power

Muscular power is the ability to produce both strength and speed. It involves generating a great force as rapidly as possible and is therefore characterised by explosive movements. It is developed by lifting near maximal weights (a weight heavy enough to allow 1–5 repetitions) very rapidly (see p. 134) and is an important aspect of performance for most sports.

MUSCLE ACTIONS

Concentric muscle actions

These occur when a muscle shortens during contraction. Examples of concentric actions include the upward phase of a biceps curl and the upward phase of a bench press.

Eccentric muscle actions

These are the reverse of a concentric action – they return the muscle to its original starting point. The muscle lengthens as the joint angle increases, releasing under controlled tension. Examples of eccentric actions include the downward phase of a biceps curl and the lowering phase of a bench press.

Isometric muscle actions

These occur when the muscle develops tension without changing its length. For example, an isometric contraction develops during a biceps curl if you cannot continue the movement beyond the mid-point – the tension in your biceps equals the resistance of the barbell.

Prime mover/agonist

The muscle that brings about a movement is called the *prime mover* or *agonist*. For example, during a biceps curl, the prime mover is the biceps muscle.

Antagonist

The muscle that acts in opposition to the prime mover, which may slow it down or stop the movement, is called the *antagonist*. It helps to keep the joint stable, and during most movements it is relaxed, allowing the movement to be performed efficiently. For example, during a biceps curl the triceps acts as the antagonist and needs to be relaxed to allow the arm to be flexed smoothly.

Synergist

A muscle that assists indirectly in a movement is called a *synergist*. For example, in a biceps curl the muscles of the forearm act as synergists because they cross the elbow joint and help to bring about the movement.

MUSCLE STRUCTURE

Muscles make up about 45 per cent of the average person's weight. They are 80 per cent water; the rest is mostly protein. Each muscle is made up of cylindrical fibres (sometimes called muscle cells), which are about 50–100 micrometres in diameter (the width of a human hair). They range from a few centimetres in length to 1 m, and can run the entire length of the muscle. These fibres are grouped in bundles called fasciculi, each separately wrapped in a sheath (perimysium) that holds them together.

Each muscle fibre comprises thread-like strands called myofibrils, each of which is about 1 micrometre in diameter, or $\frac{1}{100}$th the diameter of a human hair. These hold myofilaments containing the contractile proteins myosin (thick filaments) and actin (thin filaments), whose actions are responsible for muscle contraction (see Figure 2.1). To a large extent, your muscle's cross-sectional area, together with the number and length of its fibres, determine its strength. You cannot change the number of fibres in your muscle, but you can increase both its cross-sectional areas through strength training, as well as the number of muscle fibres recruited when executing any given movement.

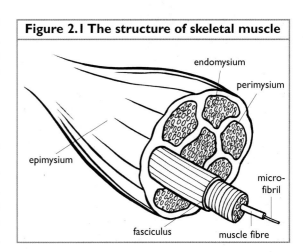

Figure 2.1 The structure of skeletal muscle

endomysium

perimysium

epimysium

micro-fibril

fasciculus

muscle fibre

MUSCLE FIBRE TYPES

Your muscle fibres can be divided into two main types:
1. slow-twitch (ST), or type I, fibres
2. fast-twitch (FT), or type II, fibres.

ST fibres are used for endurance activities. They contract relatively slowly, produce less tension and prefer to use oxygen to produce energy (i.e. aerobic metabolism). They have many capillaries and mitochondria (the powerhouses of cells) and can easily make use of both fat and carbohydrate for fuel. ST fibres do not tire easily so are used for low-intensity, long-duration aerobic activities such as walking and jogging.

FT fibres are essentially the opposite. They are best suited to anaerobic activities – anything requiring more than 25 per cent of your maximum strength. These fibres can generate high levels of tension, contract very rapidly but have poor endurance.

FT fibres can be further subdivided into FTa (type IIa) and FTb (type IIb) fibres, based on their ability to produce energy under aerobic conditions. FTa fibres have more capillaries surrounding them, more mitochondria and a greater number of aerobic enzymes than FTb fibres and, therefore, are more resistant to fatigue. The FTb fibres have the highest anaerobic capacity but the lowest endurance capacity of all fibre types. They tire very quickly and are used almost exclusively for explosive power activities such as sprinting and jumping.

Each muscle has a mix of FT and ST fibres, and this mix is largely genetically determined. Whether a muscle fibre is FT or ST is determined before birth and in the first few years of life. After this time there is little you can do to change the number or structure of your muscle fibres. Some people are born with a predominance of FT fibres, which makes them better suited to activities requiring speed, strength or power.

Can you change your muscle fibres?

It is possible to change the function of certain muscle fibre types through specific kinds of training. With aerobic training, FTa fibres can learn to use more oxygen and so assume some of the characteristics of ST fibres – i.e. they become more aerobic – while FTb fibres begin to assume some of the characteristics of FTa fibres and gain greater endurance. So, endurance training does not change the fibre type but will increase the muscles' aerobic capacity. It is not, however, possible for changes to occur in the opposite direction – i.e. for ST fibres to assume the characteristics of FT fibres.

Put simply, a top sprinter or weightlifter would probably have a high percentage of explosive FT fibres and fewer ST fibres, while an endurance athlete is more likely to have a high percentage of ST fibres and fewer FT fibres.

Regardless of your genetically determined fibre mix, you can still increase muscle size and strength through intensive training and good nutrition.

Muscle fibres and strength training

When you lift light weights – for example, during your warm-up sets or during a weight training circuit – your ST fibres carry out most of the work. As you increase the weight lifted, an increasing number of FTa and FTb fibres are also recruited. When you lift very heavy or maximal weights, both ST and FTa fibres, and virtually all of the FTb fibres are recruited. The recruitment of different fibre types as the intensity of exercise (i.e. weight lifted) increases is shown in Figure 2.2.

So, if you perform mostly light, high-repetition training, you will stimulate mostly ST fibres and

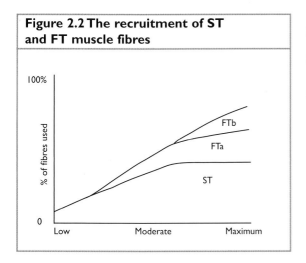

Figure 2.2 The recruitment of ST and FT muscle fibres

The all or nothing principle – a muscle fibre either contracts or it doesn't; and, when it does, it contracts with maximal force.

The size principle – as training load increases, progressively more muscle fibres are activated.

develop good muscular endurance but limited strength and size. If you incorporate both medium- and low-repetition training (i.e. using moderate and heavy weights) into your programme (bodybuilding), you will stimulate all three fibre types and therefore develop good strength, size and muscular endurance. If you perform only heavy, low-repetition training (maximal strength training), you will mainly stimulate the FTb fibres and develop good strength and moderate size, but poor muscular endurance.

HOW MUSCLES WORK

Your muscles are connected to your nervous system. They are fired, or activated, by motor nerves, and a single motor nerve may stimulate anywhere between one and several hundred muscle fibres. A nerve cell and a muscle fibre are called a *motor unit*. When a motor nerve is stimulated it causes all of the muscles fibres to contract. This is the *all or nothing principle* (see box).

The number of motor units involved in a contraction depends on the load imposed on the muscle. With a light load (weight), only a few motor units – those activating the ST fibres – are

pulled into action. As the load increases, progressively more motor units will be recruited – activating the FT fibres – until, with a maximal weight, all (or almost all) of the motor units will be recruited. Therefore, to stimulate the whole muscle, you have to work with weights that require an all-out effort. Otherwise, the highest threshold motor units never get recruited.

Muscle contraction can be explained by the *sliding filament theory of muscle contraction*. This involves the two contractile proteins, actin and myosin. When an impulse from a motor nerve reaches the muscle fibre, it creates chemical changes that cause the actin filaments to slide inwards on the myosin filaments. The myosin filaments contain cross-bridges – which are tiny extensions that reach towards the actin filaments. The myosin binds to the actin via these cross-bridges, causing them to swivel and pull the myosin filaments over the actin filaments (see Figure 2.3). This sliding is what causes the

Why do some people gain strength and muscle size more easily than others?

One explanation is that they have a greater number of muscle fibres in each motor unit. The number of fibres per motor unit is genetically determined and varies between 20 and 500, but averages around 200. So, if you have above-average fibre numbers in each motor unit, you can generate a greater force output compared to the average person. This creates a bigger stimulus for muscle growth, so your gains in strength and size will be faster.

muscle to shorten and thicken – or contract. Once the stimulation stops, the actin and myosin filaments move apart and the muscle returns to its resting length and thickness.

The force generated by the muscle depends on the weight lifted and its original length before

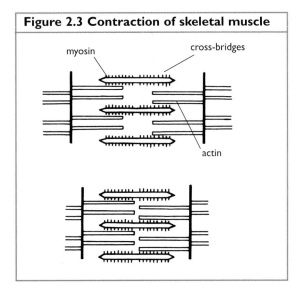

Figure 2.3 Contraction of skeletal muscle

myosin

cross-bridges

actin

contraction. If it is in its normal resting length, or slightly longer (slightly stretched), all of the cross-bridges on the myosin can connect with the actin filaments, creating greater force. For example, during a biceps curl, you will generate maximal force in the biceps muscle by starting with your arms in the fully straightened position. Starting with your arms slightly flexed will reduce the force developed and therefore the training stimulus, irrespective of the weight lifted.

HOW MUSCLES GROW

Increases in strength are the combined result of changes in the way nerve pathways serve the motor units – *neuromuscular adaptations* – and developing bigger muscles – *hypertrophy*.

When you begin lifting weights, most of the strength gains come from the nerves controlling the muscle-firing pattern becoming more efficient. The nervous system adapts to a progressive overload by improving its ability to recruit additional muscle fibres and generate more force. The greater the number of motor units involved, the greater the force of contraction. In fact, your strength gains during the first six to eight weeks of starting a strength training programme are due mostly to neuromuscular adaptation. Don't be put off if you don't get bigger muscles after the first couple of months of training. Your nervous system adapts to the new stimulus first, allowing you to maximise your strength with the muscle you already have. This is called *neuromuscular adaptation.*

After this initial period, your muscles start to grow in size and this contributes to your strength gains. The repeated contraction of muscles during weight training causes damage in the muscle tissue. The muscle proteins (actin and myosin) undergo micro-trauma – microscopic tears occur in the muscle fibres and connective tissue. This occurs primarily during the eccentric phase of the motion (see pp. 6–7) and causes the soreness you feel for a few days after an intense workout. During the rest period between workouts, new proteins are built up, the connective tissue is

Hypertrophy

Training forces your muscles to do extra work than normal to overcome the load. This process is called *overloading* and leads to increases in muscle strength and size through a process called hypertrophy.

Neuromuscular adaptation

Changes in the way nerve pathways serve the motor units are called *neuromuscular adaptation*. It's a type of motor learning – your body learns to assign more and more motor units to the movements and so you get stronger.

repaired, the muscle fibres enlarge, and the muscle increases in diameter and strength.

The increase in muscle size – *hypertrophy* – is due to an increase in the cross-sectional area of the individual fibres, rather than an increase in the number of fibres (*hyperplasia*).[1,2,3] This is the result of an increase in actin and myosin,[4] and an increase in the number of filaments within the fibres.[5] The new filaments are added in layers to the outside of the existing bundles of filaments. Thus each muscle fibre becomes denser and bigger, enlarging the whole muscle and increasing its strength.

The FT fibres increase in size more readily and at a faster rate than ST fibres.[6] Therefore, it is the growth of FT fibres that results in an increase in muscle mass and strength.[7]

Lifting weights also causes an increase in the number of blood vessels in the muscle. This means that more oxygen, fuel and nutrients can be delivered to the muscles and metabolic waste products can be removed more readily. The overall result is one of increased efficiency, strength and size.

The attached tendons, ligaments and bones also increase in strength, and so the whole surrounding structural framework becomes stronger.

Another key factor in muscle growth is improved coordination. The ability to coordinate specific movements can only be learned through practice. To perform an efficient lift, you need to relax the antagonistic muscles, so that unnecessary movement does not affect the force of the prime movers (see below). A well-coordinated group of muscles will be able to achieve a greater training effect and, therefore, better strength gains.

FACTORS AFFECTING MUSCLE MASS

The amount of muscle mass you can expect to gain will be determined by your genetic make-up, your training programme and your diet. You cannot change your genes, but by understanding your personal limitations you can work out your real strengths and weaknesses and set realistic goals. The following four factors will help you to decide your natural potential for muscle growth.

Muscle tone

Muscle tone refers to the relative state of contraction during rest. When you begin training, there is an increase in muscle tone – your muscles feel tighter – due to an increase in the packing density of the filaments.

The muscle becomes stronger and firmer to the touch in the relaxed state. This is what is commonly called 'good muscle tone'. If you don't increase your training level but maintain the same volume, the muscles do not continue to adapt so you will simply stay toned and will not increase in size. If you were to increase your training level (i.e. training volume and intensity), your muscles would increase in size as well as density.

1. Body type

Your body type dictates your genetic potential to add muscle or fat (see pp. 199–201). If you have a naturally slender frame with a small musculature (*ectomorphic* body type), your muscle gains will be slower and, ultimately, smaller than someone with a naturally athletic frame (*mesomorphic* body type). Chances are you will never closely resemble a heavyweight bodybuilder but, with hard work in the gym, you could achieve more of a lifeguard's physique. If you have a naturally large, stocky frame with a fair amount of body fat (*endomorphic* body type), you will gain muscle readily but will need to work harder with your cardiovascular training and cut back your calorie intake in order for your muscles to show. You may not achieve the sharp definition of a world-class 100 m sprinter but you could achieve the impressive muscle bulk and athleticism of a rugby player. If you are fortunate enough to be blessed with broad shoulders, narrow waist and hips and low body fat (mesomorph), you could achieve the perfect symmetry of a champion bodybuilder!

2. Muscle fibre mix

You probably have a rough idea of your mix of fast-twitch (FT) and slow-twitch (ST) muscle fibres from your natural sporting ability. If you tend to do well at sports requiring a lot of strength, speed and power, you probably have a high ratio of FT to ST fibres and will tend to gain muscle size relatively fast. On the other hand, if you tend to perform better in endurance activities, you probably have a higher proportion of ST fibres and will make slower muscle size gains. Since FT muscle fibres have the highest capacity for hypertrophy, you will experience greater gains if you have a high proportion of these.

3. Motor units

The arrangement of your motor units – the number of muscle fibres activated by each motor nerve – determines your rate of progress too. People who tend to gain strength and size very rapidly probably have an above-average number of muscle fibres in each motor unit. For the same effort, they generate a higher force output than the average person. This creates a bigger stimulus for muscle growth.

4. Hormonal balance

Your natural hormonal balance will affect your degree of muscularity and how fast you can add muscle. If you have naturally high levels of anabolic hormones such as testosterone and growth hormone (GH), you will respond to a strength training programme more readily, and achieve greater gains in muscle mass and strength than more average people. This explains why women generally never achieve the muscle bulk and strength of men, despite heavy training, as they have only one-tenth of the testosterone levels. Only by taking anabolic steroids can they achieve more masculine proportions.

The bottom line . . .

Even if you have few of these genetically determined factors on your side, you can still make great gains by paying extra attention to the quality of your training and your eating plan. Regardless of your body type, muscle fibre-type mix, motor unit make-up and hormonal level, you can improve your physique beyond measure by following a well-planned training and nutrition programme.

Realistic expectations

Most men can expect to gain 0.5–1 kg/month on an established programme.[8] Women usually experience about 50–75 per cent of the gains of men – i.e. 0.25–0.75 kg/month – partly due to their smaller initial body weight and smaller muscle mass, and partly due to lower levels of anabolic hormones.

Your weight gain may be as much as 2 kg/month during the first few months of starting strength training. In fact, lean mass gains of 20 per cent of your starting body weight are common after the first year of training. But, after a few years, you may struggle to gain 0.5 kg/month. For example, if you weigh 70 kg at the start of your training programme, you could weigh as much as 76 kg after the first three months. This would then probably drop to about 1 kg/month, so after the first year you may weigh 85 kg – that's a gain of 15 kg. Don't expect to continue adding 6–12 kg a year every year, though. Your rate of weight gain will gradually drop off over the years as you approach your genetic potential. Also, the chances are you will have temporary and unavoidable breaks from your training programme – when you go on holiday or stop training due to illness, for example. Remember, your exact rate of weight gain will be influenced by your genetic potential. That's why two people can gain very different amounts of weight despite following the same training and eating programme. If you are putting on more than 3–4 kg/month, you are probably adding body fat, so you will need to cut down on your calorie intake.

SUMMARY OF KEY POINTS

- Muscles are made up of cylindrical fibres, which comprise bundles of filaments that hold the muscle proteins.
- The proportion of FT and ST muscle fibres influences your ability to develop strength, muscle mass and endurance.
- When a muscle contracts, the two contractile proteins, actin and myosin, slide across each other to shorten the muscle.

- Strength is the combined result of hypertrophy (increase in muscle size) and neuromuscular adaptation.
- Muscles increase in strength and mass when they are subjected to progressive overload.
- An increase in muscle size is due to an increase in muscle fibre size and density rather than an increase in the number of fibres.
- The amount of lean weight you can gain depends on your genetic make-up, your natural body type, your mix of FT and ST muscle fibres, the arrangement of the motor units in your muscles and your hormonal balance, as well as the quality of your training and diet.
- Men can expect to gain 0.5–1 kg body weight/month; women can expect to gain 0.25–0.75 kg/month.
- Gains in the first year of training may be up to 20 per cent of starting body weight, then gradually slow down over the years.

MENU FOR MUSCLE

Good nutrition is a crucial part of a strength training programme. Training with weights provides the stimulus; your diet provides the raw materials for building muscle. Eating the right foods will increase your energy, maximise your gains in the gym and improve your health. It will also provide the fuel and fluid needed for intense training, speed your recovery after training, reduce fatigue and help you achieve a healthy body composition.

EAT ENOUGH

The most important thing when it comes to building muscle is calories. To gain weight, you need to take in more calories than you burn. Scientists recommend increasing your usual calorie intake by 20 per cent, which works out at about 500–750 extra calories for men and 250–500 extra calories for women. These calories should come from a balanced intake of carbohydrate, protein and fat.

HOW MANY CALORIES?

1. Food diary

Record your food intake for seven days. Be as accurate as possible, recording the exact weights of all foods and drinks consumed. Use food tables, the Internet or food labels to work out your daily calorie intake. Add up all seven days and divide by seven to get a daily average. To gain weight, add 20 per cent to that number (multiply by 1.2). This will be your new calorie intake to start adding muscle.

2. Calculation based on body weight and activity

1. Estimate your resting metabolic rate (RMR) using the appropriate equation in Table 3.1. This is the number of calories you burn at rest over 24 hours maintaining essential functions such as respiration, digestion and brain function.

Table 3.1	Resting metabolic rate in athletes[2]	
Age (years)	Men	Women
10–18	(body weight in kg x 17.5) + 651	(body weight in kg x 12.2) + 746
19–30	(body weight in kg x 15.3) + 679	(body weight in kg x 14.7) + 496
31–60	(body weight in kg x 11.6) + 879	(body weight in kg x 8.7) + 829

Example
>For a 28-year-old 70 kg male:
>RMR = (70 x 15.3) + 679 = 1750 kcal

2. Calculate your lifestyle daily energy needs based on your daily activity level, using the information below.

Daily activity level	Lifestyle daily energy needs
mostly seated or standing	RMR x 1.4
regular brisk walking or equivalent	RMR x 1.7
generally physically active	RMR x 2.0

Example
For a 28-year-old 70 kg male who is mostly sedentary:
Daily energy needs (without exercise)
>= 1750 x 1.4
>= 2450 kcal

3. Estimate your exercise calorie expenditure over a week (see Table 3.2), then divide this

Table 3.2	Calories expended during exercise	
Sport	*Kcal per hour*	
	Men	Women
Cycling (11.2 kph)	300	234
Cycling (16 kph)	450	354
Rowing machine	480	377
Running (12 kph)	840	660
Running (16 kph)	1092	858
Swimming (crawl, 4.8 kph)	1200	942
Tennis (singles)	426	330
Weight training	492	384

by seven to get a daily average. Add to your daily calorie needs. This is your total daily energy need (maintenance calorie need).

Example
For a 28-year-old 70 kg man, mostly sedentary, who spends 3 hours/week weight training and 1 hour/week running:
No. of calories burned during exercise/week = (3 x 492) + 840
>= 2316 kcal
Total daily energy needs (maintenance calorie need)
>= 2450 + (2316 ÷ 7)
>= 2781 kcal

4. **To gain weight**, increase your calorie intake by 20 per cent. Multiply your maintenance calories by 1.2.

Example
For a 28-year-old 70 kg man, mostly sedentary, who spends 3 hours/week weight training and 1 hour/week running:
Daily energy needs to gain weight
>= 2781 x 1.2
>= 3337 kcal

5. **To lose weight**, reduce your calorie intake by 15 per cent. Multiply your maintenance calories by 0.85.

Example
For a 28-year-old 70 kg man, mostly sedentary, who spends 3 hours/week weight training and 1 hour/week running:
Daily energy needs to lose weight
>= 2781 x 0.85
>= 2364 kcal

BALANCE YOUR DIET

Aim to include the suggested number of portions of each food group each day, as noted in Table 3.3 overleaf.

Table 3.3	Recommended daily portions for each food group		
Food group	**Number of portions each day**	**Food**	**Portion size**
Vegetables	3–5	I portion = 80 g	
		Broccoli, cauliflower	2–3 spears/florets
		Carrots	I carrot
		Peas	3 tablespoons
		Other vegetables	3 tablespoons
		Tomatoes	5 cherry tomatoes
Fruit	2–4	I portion = 80 g	
		Apple, pear, peach, banana	I medium fruit
		Plum, kiwi fruit, satsuma	I–2 fruit(s)
		Strawberries	8–10
		Grapes	12–16
		Tinned fruit	3 tablespoons
		Fruit juice	I medium glass
Grains and potatoes	4–6	Bread	2 slices
		Rolls/muffins	I roll
		Pasta or rice	6 tablespoons
		Breakfast cereal	I bowl
		Potatoes, sweet potatoes, yams	I fist-sized
Calcium-rich foods	2–4	Milk (dairy or calcium-fortified soya milk)	I medium cup
		Cheese	Size of 4 dice
		Tofu	Size of 4 dice
		Tinned sardines	I–2 tablespoons
		Yoghurt/fromage frais	I pot
Protein-rich foods	2–4	Lean meat	I–2 slices (40–80 g)
		Poultry	2 medium slices/I breast
		Fish	I fillet
		Egg	2
		Lentils/beans	Size of your palm
		Tof burgu/soyaer or sausage	I–2

Table 3.3	continued		
Healthy fats	I	Nuts and seeds	I heaped tablespoon
and oils		Seed oils, nut oils	I tablespoon
		Avocado	Half avocado
		Oily fish*	Size of deck of cards

* Oily fish is very rich in essential fats so just one portion a week would cover your needs.

Cutting your calorie intake

To reduce your body fat, cut your calories by 15 per cent. This relatively modest decrease minimises any drop in your metabolic rate and allows you to retain your hard-earned muscle.

The problem with drastically restricting your calorie intake is that you cause your metabolic rate to slow down. This is called the 'starvation adaptation response' and means that your body stockpiles fat and calories rather than burning them for energy so that it becomes harder and harder for your body to burn fat. Your glycogen stores also quickly deplete, causing fatigue, a drop in performance, low energy levels and mounting hunger. Worse still, you end up breaking down muscle tissue as well as fat to provide fuel. On the other hand, cutting your calories by a modest 15 per cent will produce steady fat loss without sacrificing muscle. You can expect to lose roughly 0.5 kg fat/week, slightly more when combined with the cardiovascular training programme described in Chapter 22.

Weight-gain eating tips

- Put more total eating time into your daily routine. This may mean rescheduling other activities. Plan your meal and snack times in advance and never skip or rush them, no matter how busy you are.
- Increase your meal frequency – eat at least three meals and three snacks daily.
- Eat regularly – every two to three hours – and avoid gaps longer than three hours.
- Plan nutritious high-calorie low-bulk snacks – e.g. shakes, smoothies, yoghurt, nuts, dried fruit, energy/protein bars.
- Eat larger meals but avoid overfilling!
- If you are finding it hard to eat enough food, have more drinks, such as meal replacement or protein supplements, once or twice a day to help bring up your calorie, carbohydrate and protein intake.
- Boost the calorie and nutritional content of your meals – e.g. add dried fruit, bananas, honey, chopped nuts or seeds to breakfast cereal or yoghurt. This is more nutritious than the common practice of adding sugar or jam ('empty calories').

CARBOHYDRATE

How much?

Carbohydrate, in the form of muscle glycogen and blood glucose, is the major source of fuel for strength training. Eating too little carbohydrate results in low muscle glycogen levels, low energy, reduced training intensity and fatigue. Carbohydrate also stimulates the release of insulin – an anabolic hormone that drives protein and carbohydrates into the muscle cells, encouraging muscle building. A low-carbohydrate intake causes protein breakdown and loss of muscle mass.

On the other hand, eating too much carbohydrate in one meal or over the course of a day may result in unwanted body fat once the body's glycogen storage capacity is exceeded. As a general guideline, you should consume 5–7 g carbohydrate/kg body weight/day, depending on your individual metabolism, body fat level and training volume.[1] If you weigh 75 kg, you would need a minimum of 375 g and a maximum of 525 g carbohydrate daily.

Example

For a 75 kg male:

Carbohydrate needs = (75 x 5)–(75 x 7)
= 375–525 g/day.

Calculating carbohydrate needs

The International Conference on Foods, Nutrition and Performance in 1991 recommended that carbohydrates provide 60–70 per cent of daily calories for most athletes.[1] For strength athletes, it is more accurate to calculate carbohydrate requirement according to the muscles' needs rather than total calorie intake. Muscle glycogen is not depleted the same extent as that of endurance athletes and there is longer recovery time between working the same muscle group. Carbohydrate needs are more accurately expressed as grams per kg of body weight and hours of training.[2]

Figure 3.1 The Glycaemic Index of selected high GI foods (60–100)

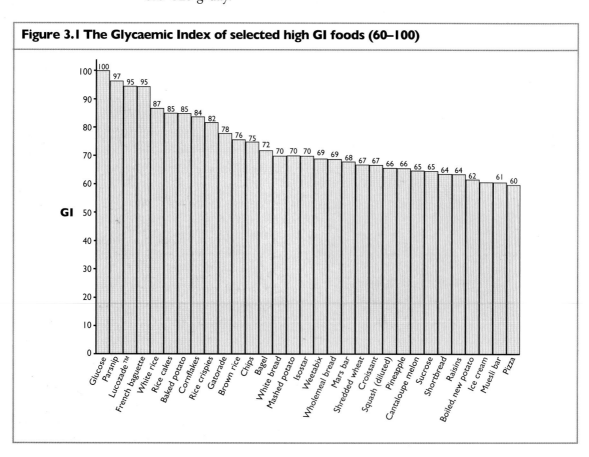

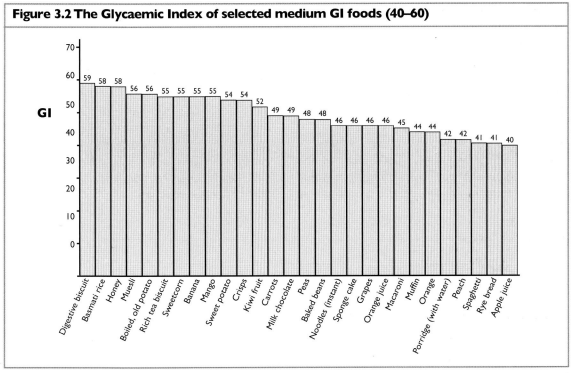

Figure 3.2 The Glycaemic Index of selected medium GI foods (40–60)

Figure 3.3 The Glycaemic Index of selected low GI foods (0–40)

Which foods?

Choose mostly fibre-rich carbohydrates like potatoes, bread, porridge, rice, pasta, fruit, beans and lentils. Honey, dried fruit and fruit juice are denser sources of carbohydrates and make it easier to reach your daily carbohydrate needs if you have a fast metabolism. If you tend to gain body fat easily or have a slower metabolism, stick with natural fibre-rich carbs, which are more filling.

Low-GI diets (see figures 3.1–3.3 for more information) are beneficial for strength trainers as well as the general population. They can help control blood sugar levels, appetite and body weight, lower blood fats, reduce the risk of diabetes and heart disease, and control body weight.[3] For strength trainers a low-GI daily diet is particularly important for encouraging glycogen recovery between workouts. It produces more steady blood glucose and insulin levels, which facilitates a steady uptake of glucose by the muscle cells for glycogen storage, and minimises the conversion of blood glucose into body fat.

The best way to plan a low-GI diet is to balance each meal by including:

- a lean source of protein (e.g. chicken breast or cottage cheese)
- a fibre-rich carbohydrate (e.g. potatoes or pasta)
- vegetables (e.g. broccoli or green salad)
- a little unsaturated fat (e.g. olive oil dressing or nuts).

The glycaemic index

The glycaemic index (GI) is a measure of how quickly your blood glucose will rise after eating a specific amount of a given carbohydrate. All foods containing carbohydrate are ranked on an index from 0 to 100 relative to pure glucose, which has the highest GI value of 100. Thus, high-GI foods produce a relatively rapid rise in blood glucose and low-GI foods produce a slower, more sustained rise in blood glucose. Figures 3.1–3.3 show the GIs of various foods, divided into high-, medium- and low-GI foods.

According to this index, many complex carbohydrates – such as potatoes, bread and rice – give a quick rise in blood glucose, while many simple carbohydrates – such as fruit – give a slower rise. It is important to realise, however, that the GI values relate to single foods being consumed. When two or more foods are eaten together, the GI changes. High GI foods eaten with protein or fat moderate the glucose response, so the GI values only count for single foods. For example, potatoes cause a relatively rapid blood glucose rise. But if you eat the potatoes with a high-protein food (e.g. tuna) or a high-fat food (e.g. butter), the resulting GI will be lower and so your blood glucose will rise more slowly.

Is carbohydrate loading beneficial for bodybuilders?

Competitive bodybuilders sometimes use carbohydrate loading to increase muscle size before a competition. Whether this really is beneficial is debatable. In one study, researchers measured the muscle girth of nine male bodybuilders before and after a control and a high-carbohydrate diet.[4] This carbohydrate-loading diet involved three days of heavy weight training on a low-carbohydrate diet (10 per cent calories from carbohydrate), followed by three days of light weight training on a high-carbohydrate diet (80 per cent calories from carbohydrate). The control diet involved the same weight training programme but the men ate a standard diet providing the same number of calories. So what happened? Carbohydrate loading did not increase the muscle circumference in any of the bodybuilders, which suggests that it probably has no benefit after all.

Obviously, this is just a single study so its findings are not conclusive. There is plenty of anecdotal evidence from bodybuilders that carbohydrate loading before a competition improves muscle appearance. If you decide to try this regime, however, you may achieve equally good results by omitting the three-day depletion phase and simply eating a high-carbohydrate diet for the three days prior to competition.

PROTEIN

How much?

Protein is important for muscle growth. Heavy strength training stimulates an increased uptake of amino acids from the bloodstream. These amino acids are then built up into new contractile muscle proteins, actin and myosin (see p. 7). To build muscle, you must take in more protein than you excrete – i.e. be in a positive nitrogen balance. A deficiency will result in slower gains in strength, size and mass, or even muscle loss – despite hard training. However, there is not a linear relationship between protein intake and muscle growth. Muscle growth depends not only on your protein intake but also on the intensity of your training (i.e. the training stimulus) and your genetic potential for muscle growth.

In practice the body can adapt to variations in protein intake. Over time the body becomes more efficient in conserving it so you break down fewer muscle proteins during intense training. This is often sufficient to maintain an anabolic environment and induce muscle growth.[5] One study found that the protein requirement/kg body weight of advanced strength trainers was 40 per cent less than that of novice strength trainers.[6]

It is generally recommended that strength trainers need 1.4–1.8 g/kg body weight/day[5,6] compared with the recommended daily allowance (RDA) of 0.75 g/kg body weight/day for the general population. A 75 kg male would need between (75 x 1.4) = 105 g and (75 x 1.8) = 135 g per day.

Divide your protein intake into five or six meals spaced every three to four hours. Aim to include 20–25 g protein in each of your meals. Eating this way maximises protein absorption and minimises fat storage.

Too much protein?

Consuming more than 1.8 g protein/kg body weight/day will not make you stronger or more muscular.[7] In a study of strength athletes carried out at McMaster University, Ontario, athletes consuming either 1.4 g/kg body weight/day or 2.3 g/kg body weight/day experienced similar increases in muscle mass.[5] Those with the higher protein intake gained no further benefits. Once your optimal intake has been reached, additional protein is not converted into muscle.

Table 3.4	The protein content of various foods	
Food	**Portion size**	**Protein (g)**
Meat and fish		
Beef – fillet steak, grilled	105 g	31
Chicken breast – grilled, meat only	130 g	39
Turkey – light meat, roasted	140 g	47
Cod – poached	120 g	25
Mackerel – grilled	150 g	31
1 small tin tuna – canned in brine	100 g	24
Dairy products		
Cheese, cheddar (1 thick slice)	40 g	10
1 small carton cottage cheese	112 g	15
1 glass skimmed milk	200 ml	7
1 carton low-fat yoghurt – fruit	150 g	6
Eggs (size 2)	1	8
Nuts and seeds		
Peanuts – roasted and salted (handful)	50 g	10
Peanut butter on 1 slice bread	20 g	5
Cashew nuts – roasted and salted (handful)	50 g	10
2 tbsp sesame seeds	24 g	4
Pulses		
1 small tin baked beans	205 g	10
3 tbsp red lentils – boiled	120 g	9
3 tbsp red kidney beans – boiled	120 g	10
Soya and Quorn products		
2 tbsp dry soya mince	30 g	13
Tofu burger	60 g	5
4 tbsp Quorn mince	100 g	12
Grains and cereals		
2 slices wholemeal bread	76 g	6
1 bowl pasta – boiled	230 g	7

Protein and amino acids

There are dozens of amino acids but the body uses only 20 of them as the building blocks of proteins. Eight of these are 'indispensable amino acids' (IAAs) – that is, they are essential and must be supplied in the diet as the body cannot make them itself. The remaining 12 can be made from other amino acids and are termed 'dispensable' – in other words, they are non-essential.

Three IAAs – valine, leucine and isoleucine – are termed BCAAs, due to their branched structure. These are used as fuel for energy by the muscles during intense exercise when glycogen stores are low. Food proteins with a high IAA content in proportions closely matched to the body's requirements are said to have a high biological value (BV). This is a measure of the usefulness of a protein – that is, the proportion of the protein that can be absorbed and used for growth and repair. Eggs have the highest BV (100) of all foods, although, according to supplement manufacturers, whey protein supplements have even higher values.

To maximise the benefits of protein in your diet, eat a mixture of protein foods so that the shortfall of amino acids in one is complemented by higher amounts in the other. For example, combining beans and rice means that the shortfall of lysine in rice is complemented by higher amounts in the beans. Other combinations suitable for vegetarians include tortillas filled with refried beans, rice with chickpeas, rice crackers with peanut butter, Quorn burger in a bun and stir-fried tofu with noodles.

Which foods?

You should get the majority of your protein from food sources rather than supplements. Animal sources (poultry, fish, meat, dairy products and eggs) generally have a higher biological value (BV) (see the box entitled 'Protein and amino acids') than plant sources (tofu, Quorn, beans, lentils, nuts and cereals). However, if you eat a mixture of animal and plant sources, you will get more amino acids as well as a better range of other nutrients (fibre, vitamins, minerals and carbohydrate).

If you're trying to gain muscle mass but want to keep body fat under control, choose lower-fat protein sources like skinless poultry, low-fat dairy products and protein powders.

The protein content of various foods is given in Table 3.4 (see p. 21).

FAT

Athletes should consume 15–30 per cent of their calories from fat.[1] Eating too little fat puts you at risk of a deficient intake of 'fat-soluble vitamins' A, D and E, and essential fatty acids.

Essential fats

The two essential fatty acids – linoleic acid and alpha-linolenic acid – are vital to your health and cannot be made in the body. When you eat linoleic acid, your body converts it into a number of other fatty acids, including gamma-linolenic acid (GLA) and docosapentanoic acid (DPA). Linoleic acid and its derivative fatty acids are called omega-6 fatty acids (there is a rigid link, or 'double bond', on the sixth carbon atom in the fatty acid chain). When you eat alpha-linolenic acid, your body converts it into eicosapentanoic acid (EPA) and docosahexanoic acid (DHA), and these are called omega-3 fatty acids (the rigid link occurs on the third carbon atom).

Both omega-6 (from most vegetable oils and margarines) and omega-3 (from oily fish and certain nuts and seeds) fatty acids are essential for good health. They are involved in cell membrane structure, especially in the retina of the eye, the brain and the heart, and the body also uses them to produce a group of hormone-like substances called 'eicosanoids'. These regulate many processes in the body, such as the inflammatory and immune responses.

How much?

There is no RDA for essential fatty acids, although the government advises eating at least one portion of oily fish per week, which will provide around 2–3 g EPA and DHA. A separate recommendation of 0.65 g EPA and DHA/day has also been made.[8] Aim to eat one to two portions of oily fish (sardines, mackerel, salmon) a week or one tablespoon of an omega-3-rich oil (e.g. walnut, flaxseed, rapeseed, pumpkin seed) daily.

For good health and performance you need to consume a balance of omega-3s and omega-6s –

at least 1 g omega-3s for every 5 g of omega-6s.[8] Most people currently consume too much omega-6s and too little omega-3s. Many experts believe that it is this imbalance of omega-3s to omega-6s that contributes to many health problems, such as heart disease, inflammation, rheumatoid arthritis and pain, even slow post-workout recovery.

Omega-3s and exercise

There is mounting evidence to suggest that consuming more omega-3s may reduce inflammation, pain and joint stiffness, and speed post-workout recovery.[9] It may also enhance aerobic performance by optimising oxygen delivery to your cells, reducing blood viscosity and making red cell membranes more flexible.

Table 3.5	The omega-3 and omega-6 fatty acid content of various foods			
Food	Portion	Omega-3s	Omega-6s	Omega-6: Omega-3 ratio
Good sources of omega-3s				
Rapeseed oil	I tbsp	I.5	3.1	1:0.49
Cod liver oil	I tbsp	2.7	0.9	1:3
Flaxseed oil	I tbsp	7.5	1.8	1:4.2
Walnut oil	I tbsp	I.4	7.5	5.3:1
Salmon	100 g	I.5	0.6	1:2.5
Herring	100 g	1.8	0.6	1:3
Trout	100 g	2	1.4	1:1.4
Omega-3 fortified egg	I	0.7	0.7	1:1
Typical fatty-acid supplement*		0.5	0.1	1:5
Good sources of omega-6s				
Corn oil	I tbsp	0.1	7.9	79:1
Soya margarine	I tbsp	0.1	3.5	25:1
Mayonnaise	I tbsp	0.4	7.2	18:1
Safflower oil	I tbsp	0.05	10.1	202:1
Soya oil	I tbsp	I	7.2	7.2:1
Goal				5:1

*8 capsules (the recommended daily dose) of 'Efalex'

Source: Simopoulos, A.P. and Robinson, J. (1998), The Omega Plan (New York: HarperCollins).

Which foods?

Oily fish – such as mackerel, pilchards, trout, salmon, herring and sardines – is the richest source of omega-3s. However, alpha-linolenic acid (the precursor to EPA and DHA) is also found in other foods – like sweet potatoes, walnuts, almonds, rapeseed oil, walnut oil, soya oil, flaxseed oil, flaxseeds, chicken and beef. Alternatively, supplements and foods fortified with omega-3s (e.g. omega-3-enriched eggs, margarine and bread) can also help increase your intake. The best sources of omega-3 and omega-6 fatty acids are given in Table 3.5 on p. 23.

EATING BEFORE TRAINING

Eating a low-GI meal two to four hours before training will produce a slower release of energy, help maintain blood sugar levels during your workout and spare muscle glycogen. Porridge, cereal with milk, a chicken or cheese sandwich, a jacket potato with beans, or pasta with tuna are suitable pre-workout meals. Combining carbohydrate with protein and/or fat gives a slower burn than carbohydrate alone. If your last meal was more than four hours before your workout, have a small carbohydrate-rich snack – a banana, a handful of dried fruit, a fruit smoothie, 300 ml of diluted fruit juice (50/50) or a sports drink – about an hour before your workout to boost blood sugar levels.

Although most of the research on pre-exercise meals has been carried out with endurance athletes, it seems that consuming approximately 1 g carbohydrate/kg body weight about an hour before exercise helps you keep going significantly longer than consuming nothing.

EATING DURING TRAINING

There is plenty of evidence from studies with endurance athletes that consuming carbohydrate during exercise lasting more than one hour maintains blood sugar levels, delays fatigue, and improves endurance and performance.[10] A few studies also suggest that consuming a carbohydrate/protein drink during a strenuous weights workout lasting 45–60 minutes may encourage faster muscle growth, delay fatigue and give you more energy to perform those last few sets. It may also reduce the risk of excessive protein (muscle) breakdown during the latter stages of your workout.

However, if you wish to lose body fat or prevent fat gain, be aware that many commercial energy drinks are high in calories. If you drink too much, you could end up taking in more calories than you burn off!

EATING AFTER TRAINING

Studies have shown that consuming carbohydrate within two hours of exercise speeds glycogen recovery[13] and improves performance the next day.[14]

Combining carbohydrate with protein seems more effective strategy for replenishing glycogen than consuming carbohydrate alone.[15,16,17,18] A study at the University of Texas at Austin found that a carbohydrate/protein shake (112 g carbohydrate plus 40 g protein) accelerated glycogen re-stocking in the muscle by 38 per cent compared with carbohydrate-only drinks.[15] Protein combined with carbohydrate stimulates a greater release of insulin, which promotes faster uptake of glucose by the muscle cells and faster glycogen storage. Protein-only drinks fail to increase muscle glycogen,[15] so save them until later or, better still, add some carbohydrate to them to make them more useful.

However, the benefits of a post-exercise carbohydrate/protein drink don't stop there. A fur-

Do workouts on an empty stomach burn more fat?

If fat loss is your main goal, exercising on an empty stomach may encourage your body to burn slightly more fat for fuel. The reason? Insulin levels are at their lowest after an overnight fast. This increases the amount of fat that leaves your fat cells and travels to your muscles, where the fat is burned. On the downside, you may fatigue sooner or drop your exercise intensity and therefore end up burning fewer calories – and less body fat! Worse, you could end up losing hard-earned muscle as you start burning protein – as well as fat – for fuel!

According to research from the Human Performance Laboratory at the University of Texas at Austin, fat burning is suppressed when carbohydrates are eaten during the six hours before exercise. This is due to the rise in insulin levels in the blood (caused by carbohydrates), which suppresses the breakdown of fat stores in adipose tissue and reduces the release of fatty acids into the bloodstream. Thus, fatty acids are less readily available as a fuel for the exercising muscles, an effect that can last for several hours after eating carbohydrates. Doing your cardio workout after a period of fasting (e.g. first thing in the morning), when blood insulin levels are relatively low, will optimise the rate of fat breakdown and fat burning, and would be a more effective fat-burning strategy than doing your cardio workout later in the day after you have eaten a few meals. However, it is more important that you fit your cardio workout comfortably into your daily schedule than risk omitting it if you are unable to fit it in during the morning.

ther study at the University of Texas at Austin found that such drinks also promote greater growth hormone (GH) release following a weights workout.[18] It seems as if the combination of higher insulin and GH levels creates an ideal anabolic (muscle-building) environment.

How workout drinks could make you stronger

Researchers at California State University gave 10 male weight trainers either a protein/carbohydrate drink or a placebo immediately before and during an intense weight training workout lasting two hours.[11] Those who had consumed the protein/carb drink maintained higher blood glucose and insulin levels throughout the workout, which, say the researchers, could promote even greater muscle growth. This is because insulin increases the uptake of amino acids into muscle cells and reduces protein breakdown – the ideal state for muscle hypertrophy. Although the workout in this study lasted longer than one hour, it is possible that carbohydrate or carbohydrate/protein drinks during a shorter workout may be beneficial too.

A study with cyclists also found that drinking a carbohydrate drink before and during a time trial lasting approximately one hour improved performance time.[12]

Carbohydrate-plus-protein also improves mood state after training. Researchers at Ithaca College, New York, carried out a psychological survey on weight trainers after consuming either a carbohydrate/protein drink or meal, a carbohydrate-only drink or a placebo drink.[19] Those who consumed the carbohydrate/protein combination, either in liquid or solid form, experienced less mental distress, less irritability and less fatigue than the others.

Aim for a balance of 1 g of protein for every 3 g of carbohydrate in your post-workout snack or drink. As fat can reduce the rate of glycogen storage, make sure your recovery snack is low in fat. Some ideas for suitable post-workout snacks are given in the box overleaf.

Post-workout snacks

- Meal-replacement shake (carbohydrate/protein drink)
- Protein shake and a banana
- Chicken sandwich
- Baked potato with cottage cheese
- Porridge made with skimmed milk
- Tuna sandwich
- Wholegrain breakfast cereal with skimmed milk and yoghurt
- Fruit yoghurt
- Protein/energy bar

EATING BETWEEN WORKOUTS

To promote efficient recovery between workouts, divide your food into several small meals – ideally all with a low GI value. Frequent small meals produce more stable blood sugar and insulin levels, promote efficient glycogen storage and increase the metabolic rate. When you eat more frequently throughout the day, you encourage your body to use calories more efficiently, rather than storing them as body fat. Every time you eat a meal, extra calories are burned to digest and metabolise the food. This is called the thermic effect of food. A mixed meal – protein, carbohydrates and fats blended together – uses about 10 per cent of the calories for this purpose. For optimal muscle-building and fat-burning effects, you should consume approximately six balanced meals or snacks throughout the day. Each meal should include one to two portions of carbohydrate-rich foods and at least one portion of a protein-rich food. Include plenty of vegetables with at least two of your daily meals, and eat a minimum of three portions of fruit each day. Table 3.6 lists nutrient-rich carbohydrate- and protein-rich foods, and gives practical advice to help you plan your daily meals.

WATER

Of all the nutrients, water is the most important. Without any water or fluid, you'll last less than a week. It makes up more than 60 per cent of your body weight and is vital to all cells.

Water is the medium in which all metabolic reactions take place, including energy production. One key fluid – blood – carries nutrients and oxygen to the cells and helps rid the body of toxins. Fluid acts as a cushion for your nervous system and acts as a lubricant for your joints and eyes. On top of that, proper hydration helps to keep your body temperature stable – you sweat when you get too hot.

You need to top up your fluid levels frequently because you lose water through sweating, breathing and urinating. Most experts recommend consuming at least a litre of water for every 1000 kcal expended. Since about one-third will come from the food you eat, the British Dietetic Association recommends drinking at least 1.5 litres/day. That's equivalent to roughly six to eight glasses, although you'll need to drink more during hot weather and when you exercise. Table 3.7 gives some tips on how to drink more water and keep properly hydrated.

Drinking and exercise

Drinking water before and during training will help you to exercise harder and longer. One of the most important roles of water is to get rid of the excess heat produced by your exercising muscles. Water from your blood and extracellular (outside the body cells) spaces is transported to the skin's surface, and evaporated by heat (sweating). If you're low on water, your muscle control and strength will diminish. A loss of just 2 per cent of your body weight can reduce your muscle strength and your aerobic capacity by at least 10 per cent. Your thirst mechanism only kicks in when you have lost 2 per cent of your

Table 3.6 — Meal planning for strength training

Protein-rich food: choose 1 portion/meal	Carb-rich food: choose 1–2 portions/meal	Vegetables: choose 3+ portions/day	Fruit: choose 3+ portions/day	Omega-3-rich fats:* choose 1–2 portions/day	Omega-6-rich fats:* choose 1/day	Sample meal combinations
Chicken breast	Potato	Broccoli	Apples	Omega-3-enriched margarine	Sunflower oil	Baked potato with omega-3 enriched margarine, grilled chicken and broccoli; stewed apples
Turkey breast	Pasta	Carrots	Cherries	Cod liver oil	Corn oil	Pasta tossed with flaxseed oil; turkey and vegetable stir fry; cherries
White fish, e.g. tuna tinned in water/brine cod, haddock, plaice	Wholegrain bread	Salad leaves	Oranges/clementines/satsumas	Rapeseed oil	Olive oil	Tuna sandwich (with olive oil margarine); side salad with walnut oil dressing; oranges
Oily fish, e.g. salmon, sardines, mackerel	Rice	Cauliflower	Nectarines	Salmon	Soya oil	Baked salmon; boiled rice; cauliflower
Tofu	Noodles	Peppers	Plums	Flaxseeds	Margarine made with sunflower/soya/corn/olive oil	Noodles with stir-fried peppers and tofu; plum crumble sprinkled with flaxseeds
Low-fat cheese	Rice cakes/crackers	Tomatoes	Apricots	Mackerel	Mayonnaise made with sunflower/olive oil	Rice cakes with low-fat cheese and tomatoes; apricots
Yoghurt*	Wholegrain breakfast cereal	Brussels sprouts	Kiwi fruit	Walnuts	Nuts	Muesli with yoghurt, walnuts and almonds; kiwi fruit
Quorn	Beans and lentils*	Mangetout	Melon	Walnut oil	Sunflower seeds	Quorn and bean stew; mangetout; melon
Lean cuts of meat	Sweet potato	Spinach	Mango	Sardines	Salad dressing made with sunflower/olive oil	Grilled lean sirloin steak; sweet potato; spinach salad with dressing; mango
Milk*	Porridge oats	Cabbage	Strawberries	Pilchards		Porridge with milk; strawberries
Cottage cheese	Sweetcorn	Green beans	Papaya	Omega-3-enriched egg		Cottage cheese mixed with papaya (snack)
Egg	Milk*		Bananas	Flaxseed oil		Banana milkshake with flaxseed oil (snack)
Beans and lentils*	Yoghurt*	Onions	Grapes	Trout		Lentil dahl (with onions) topped with yoghurt

*These foods contain roughly equal amounts of protein and carbohydrate. Only count them once for each meal.

Table 3.7	How to keep hydrated

- Keep a bottle of water on your desk
- Carry a waterbottle with you throughout the day
- If you don't like the taste of tap water, try bottled water or flavour it with a slice of lemon or lime
- Other options include flavoured water and 'low calorie' soft drinks (but try to avoid those laden with artificial sweeteners and flavours), herb and fruit tea, weak tea, and coffee substitutes
- Have a 'water break' at least once an hour – set the timer on your watch to remind yourself
- Get into the habit of having a water break instead of a coffee break
- Drink water before, during and after your workout – take a 1-litre bottle of water to the gym

body weight – by which time your performance will already have suffered.

If water is not replaced during exercise, your blood volume drops, your cardiovascular system becomes stressed, your heart rate increases, your blood pressure rises and exercise feels much harder. You also begin to lose concentration and feel more tired. A 4 per cent drop in body weight due to dehydration causes a 20–30 per cent drop in strength. You may also get headaches, cramp-

ing, dizziness and nausea. Severe dehydration (8–10 per cent loss of body weight) can lead to heat stroke and death.

Dehydration check

Check the colour of your urine – the more transparent it is (i.e. the less yellow), the better hydrated you are. If it is a golden colour or a deep colour with a strong odour, you are dehydrated. Passing a small volume of urine having experienced a strong sensation to visit the toilet is also an indicator.

Thirst

Thirst is the most important mechanism for ensuring you take in enough fluid. When you experience thirst – a dry mouth and throat, a craving for drink – your body is signalling dehydration. This is detected by osmoreceptors in the hypothalamus region of your brain. They are able to detect changes in the osmotic pressure and volume of body fluids. When your body's fluid level becomes low, the sodium concentration and, therefore, osmolality of your blood rises, signalling the thirst sensation in the hypothalamus. So, you get the urge to drink.

It is important to realise that feeling thirsty is like a red flag – it means you are already dehydrated by at least 2 per cent of your body weight. You should not wait until you get into this state before topping up. To keep properly hydrated, drink before, during and after a workout.

DRINKING BEFORE, DURING AND AFTER TRAINING

Make sure you are properly hydrated before your workout. The American College of Sports Medicine (ACSM) recommends drinking 400–600 ml of fluid two to three hours before exercise[20] then 150–350 ml every 15–20 minutes during exercise. In hot or humid conditions you will lose more fluid so you will need to drink more. Make regular drink breaks a part of your workouts and start drinking early in your workout. If you wait until you are thirsty, you will become dehydrated and your performance will already have suffered by the time you drink. If you feel nauseous when you drink, this indicates that you are dehydrated, so ensure you drink plenty of water. After your workout is the time to replace any fluid you have lost. Drink 1.5 litres for every 1 kg you have lost.

Water is the best drink for replacing lost body fluids for exercise lasting less than one hour. Sports drinks containing carbohydrate and sodium also replace fluid rapidly, but are more beneficial for intense exercise lasting longer than one hour. Most contain 4–8 g carbohydrate/100 ml, and are designed to help maintain blood glucose levels and combat fatigue when muscle glycogen levels run low. It is possible that they may help you do a few more repetitions or sets at the end of your workout if you are training for longer than one hour but, so far, there have not been any studies on the benefits of sports drinks on strength training exercise lasting less than one hour.

VITAMINS AND MINERALS

Getting the right balance of vitamins and minerals is important not only for good health but also for your performance in the gym. Regular heavy strength training places additional demands on your body that increase your requirement for many vitamins and minerals, higher than the RDAs set for the general population. Coupled with busy lifestyles, erratic eating habits or calorie-restricted diets, many athletes end up with vitamin and mineral intakes below the RDAs.[21] This could leave you lacking in energy, failing to make gains in size and strength, susceptible to minor infections and illnesses, or at risk of more serious conditions such as stress fractures and anaemia. Table 3.8 summarises the exercise-related functions, best food sources and requirements of 12 key vitamins and minerals.

Five a day

The government and the World Health Organization recommend eating at least five portions of fruit and vegetables (equivalent to 400 g) a day. Try to consume two to four portions of fruit and three to five portions of vegetables – the more intensely coloured the better. Table 3.9 shows the healthiest fruit and vegetables, ranked by researchers at Tuft's University for their ability to soak up free radicals. Fruit and vegetables are rich in vitamins – especially vitamin C and beta-carotene, minerals, fibre and important plant nutrients, which help protect against heart disease and cancer, and boost your immunity.

ANTIOXIDANTS

Antioxidants are substances that quench free radicals. They include enzymes, vitamins (such as beta-carotene, and vitamins C and E), minerals (such as selenium and zinc) and plant substances called phytochemicals. The body produces free radicals all the time but they are increased during exercise (as well as exposure to cigarette smoke, pollutants and ultra-violet light). This is due to the 10–20-fold increase in oxygen consumption, the increase in lactic acid production and the increase in heat generation. Intense weight training also results in micro-tears in the muscle that generate more free radicals, and this is partly responsible for post-exercise soreness and tenderness.

The body tends to adapt – thankfully – by producing higher levels of antioxidant enzymes to deal with the additional amount of free radicals.

Table 3.8	The essential guide to vitamins and minerals				
Vitamin/ mineral	RNI and USL*	Major functions	Why strength trainers may need more	Best food sources	Dangers of high doses
Carotenoids	• No official RNI: 15 mg beta-carotene suggested • USL = 100 mg	• Vision in dim light • Healthy skin • Converts into vitamin A	Exercise increases need for antioxidants. Antioxidants may protect against certain cancers and reduce muscle soreness	• Intensely coloured fruit and vegetables e.g. apricots, peppers, tomatoes, mangoes, broccoli	Excessive doses of beta-carotene can cause harmless (and reversible) orange tinge to skin
Thiamin	• RNI = 0.4 mg/1000 kcal • USL = 20 mg	• Converts carbo-hydrates to energy	To process the extra carbohydrates eaten	• Wholemeal bread and cereals • Pulses • Meat	Excess is excreted, so toxicity is rare
Riboflavin	• RNI = 1.3 mg (men); 1.1 mg (women) • USL = 200 mg	• Converts carbo-hydrates to energy	To process the extra carbohydrates eaten	• Milk and dairy products • Meat • Eggs	Excess is excreted (producing yellow urine!), so toxicity is rare
Niacin	• RNI = 6.6 mg/1000 kcal • USL = 150 mg (2 g)	• Converts carbo-hydrates to energy	To process the extra carbohydrates eaten	• Meat and offal • Nuts • Milk and dairy products • Eggs • Wholegrain bread and cereals	Excess is excreted, but high doses may cause hot flushes
Vitamin C	• RNI = 40 mg • USL = 2000 mg (2 g)	• Healthy connective tissue, bones, teeth, blood vesels, gums and teeth • Promotes immune function • Helps iron absorp-tion	Exercise increases need for antioxidants, may help reduce free radical damage, protect cell membranes and reduce post-exercise muscle soreness	• Fruit and vegetables (e.g. raspberries, blackcurrants, kiwi, oranges, peppers, broccoli, cabbage, tomatoes)	Excess is excreted, but doses over 2 g may lead to diarr-hoea and excess urine formation. High doses (> 2 g) may cause vitamin C to behave as a a pro-oxidant (enhance free radical damage)
Vitamin E	• No RNI in UK; 10 mg in EU USL = 800 mg	• Antioxidant which helps protect against heart disease • Promotes normal cell growth and development	Exercise increases need for antioxidants; may help reduce free radical damage, protect cell membranes and reduce post-exercise muscle soreness	•Vegetable oils • Margarine • Oily fish • Nuts and seeds • Egg yolk • Avocados	Toxicity is rare

Vitamin/ mineral	RNI and USL*	Major functions	Why strength trainers may need more	Best food sources	Dangers of high doses
Calcium	• RNI = 1000 mg (men); 700 mg (women) • USL = 1500 mg	• Builds bone and teeth • Blood clotting • Nerve and muscle function	Low oestrogen in female athletes with amenorrhoea increases bone loss and need for calcium	• Milk and dairy products • Sardines • Dark green leafy vegetables • Pulses • Nuts and seeds	High intakes may interfere with absorption of other minerals; take with magnesium and vitamin D
Iron	• RNI = 8.7 mg (men); 14.8 mg (women) • USL = 15 mg	• Formation of red blood cells • Oxygen transport • Prevents anaemia	Female athletes may need more to compensate for menstrual losses	• Meat and offal • Wholegrain bread and cereals • Fortified breakfast cereals • Pulses • Green leafy vegetables	Constipation, discomfort. Avoid unnecessary supplementation – may increase free radical damage
Zinc	• RNI = 9.5 mg (men); 7.0 mg (women) • USL = 15 mg	• Healthy immune system • Wound healing • Skin formation • Cell growth	Exercise increases need for antioxidants; may help immune function	• Eggs • Wholegrain cereals • Meat • Milk and dairy products	Interferes with absorption of iron and copper
Magnesium	• RNI = 300 mg (men); 270 mg (women) • USL = 300 mg	• Healthy bones • Muscle and nerve function • Cell formation	May improve recovery after strength training; increase aerobic capacity	• Cereals • Fruit and vegetables • Milk	Take with calcium and vitamin D. May cause diarrhoea
Potassium	• RNI = 3.5 mg • USL = no value	• Fluid balance • Muscle and nerve function	May help prevent cramp	• Fruit and vegetables • Cereals	Excess is excreted
Selenium	• RNI = 75 µg (men); 60 µg (women) • USL = 200 µg	• Antioxidant which helps protect against heart disease and cancer	Exercise increases free radical production	• Cereals • Vegetables • Dairy products • Meat • Eggs	Nausea, vomiting and hair loss

*RNI = Reference Nutrient Intake (Dept. of Health, 1991). This is the amount of a nutrient that should cover the needs of 97% of the population. Athletes in hard training may need more.

*USL = Upper Safe Levels for daily supplementation. It defines the intake of nutrients from supplements that could be consumed on a long-term basis. This term was used in a report issued by the European Federation of Health Product Manufacturers (EHPM) and the UK Council for Responsible Nutrition (CRN) in 1997. It is not a definition of levels that could be advocated to promote general health and should not be exceeded.

Table 3.9	The healthiest fruit and vegetables	
		ORAC Score*
Fruit		
Prunes		5770
Raisins		2830
Blueberries		2400
Blackberries		2036
Strawberries		1540
Raspberries		1220
Plums		949
Oranges		750
Red grapes		739
Cherries		670
Vegetable		
Kale		1770
Spinach		1260
Brussels sprouts		980
Broccoli		890
Beetroot		840
Red peppers		710
Onion		450
Sweetcorn		400

*Oxygen Radical Absorbance Capacity – i.e. the ability to combat harmful free radicals per 100 g.

What are free radicals?

A free radical is an atom or molecule containing an unpaired electron. It is highly unstable and reactive, and capable of damaging fat- and protein-containing tissues.

Free radicals are produced continually during normal cell processes and at low levels even have a useful role: they help manufacture prostaglandins, kill bacteria and heal wounds. It's only when free radicals are present in excessive numbers that they cause problems. They can destroy cell membranes, membrane proteins, DNA (the genetic material found in every cell), enzymes, blood cholesterol and mitochondria membranes, and over a period of time free radical damage is thought to be responsible for the development of arteriosclerosis, several cancers and the ageing process.

Some bodybuilders eat very monotonous diets, centred on only a few foods. This is bad news because the more restricted your diet is, the less likely you are to obtain all the vitamins and minerals you need. By increasing the variety of foods in your diet, you will automatically be getting more vitamins and minerals.

SUPPLEMENTS

Vitamin and mineral supplements

A multivitamin and mineral supplement can act as an insurance policy if you aren't getting enough nutrients from your food. Regard it as a top-up rather than a main provider of your intake. Supplements should not be substitutes for a badly planned diet but they may be beneficial if:

- you eat erratically and fail to consume five portions of fruit and vegetables a day
- you are on a calorie-restricted diet providing less than 1500 kcal/day
- you exclude one or more major food groups (e.g. a dairy-free diet).

Bodybuilding and vitamins

One study of competitive bodybuilders found that those who consumed roughly 1500 kcal/day had low intakes of several minerals, which put them at risk of calcium, zinc, copper and chromium deficiencies.[22] Researchers at the University of Alabama at Birmingham, Alabama, also found that competitive bodybuilders consumed less than 70% of the RDA for folic acid, vitamin E, calcium, potassium and zinc.[23] These low intakes were partly due to their low-calorie (food) intakes during the pre-competition diet, and partly due to their avoidance of dairy products.

There is little evidence that vitamin and mineral supplements enhance performance. In studies, those athletes who were given vitamin and mineral supplements for a period of eight months did not experience greater gains in strength, power or endurance compared with athletes given a placebo (dummy pill).[23,24] On the other hand, the studies did not measure the health-enhancing effects of supplements, or their effect on post-workout recovery. Given that vitamins and minerals are essential for energy production, muscle manufacture, red blood cell formation, cell division and virtually every other metabolic process, it seems logical that an adequate intake will optimise all of these processes. And a supplement may just help you achieve this. A sub-optimal intake would clearly reduce the efficiency of these processes, slow down your recovery, and have a negative effect on your performance. The whole point of taking a supplement is to ensure 'normal' levels of vitamins and minerals that will support health and performance.

Meal replacement supplements

Meal replacement supplements – shakes and bars containing protein, carbohydrate, vitamins and minerals – provide a nutritionally balanced and convenient alternative to food. Most contain whey protein, which may help meet your protein requirement, spare muscle during intense training and enhance your immune system. They are intended to be taken between meals to supplement your nutritional intake, rather than in place of meals. On the down side, they are low in fibre and may contain artificial sweeteners, flavourings and colours.

Protein supplements

Protein powders – mostly whey, casein or soy protein – basically supplement your protein intake. They can help meet your daily protein

Is it possible to overdose on supplements?

Supplements taken in excess of your requirements may be harmful in high doses. For example, regular daily doses of vitamin A greater than 1500 micrograms during pregnancy can cause birth defects in unborn babies. A single dose of 150,000 micrograms may cause weakness and vomiting.

To avoid excess doses, it is best taken in the form of beta-carotene or carotenoid supplements (these can be converted into vitamin A in the body as required). Regular daily doses of vitamin D greater than 50 micrograms can cause constipation or diarrhoea, nausea and heartbeat irregularities, and can ultimately cause calcium to accumulate in the muscles. Most supplements contain up to 10 micrograms of vitamin D. High doses of vitamin B6 (more than 2000 mg/day) can cause nerve damage if taken over a period of time. So, always check the amounts of these vitamins on the label and follow the recommended dose given by the manufacturer. The Food Standards Agency gives safe upper limits for supplements.

Avoid single-nutrient supplements – unless advised by a nutritionist or health professional – as they can result in imbalances. Many vitamins and minerals interact and work as a team. It is better to take a multivitamin formulation rather than individual supplements.

requirement and are particularly useful for those with high protein requirements who find it difficult to consume enough food. They may also be taken by those on a calorie-restricted diet (additional protein can offset muscle breakdown) or by those consuming a vegetarian or vegan diet (most plant sources contain considerably less protein per gram compared with animal sources, making it more difficult to meet the body's needs from food alone).

The pros and cons of different protein supplements are summarised in Table 3.10.

Table 3.10	Protein pros and cons		
Protein source	**Derived from**	**Pros**	**Cons**
Whey	A by-product of cheese manufacture	• Excellent ratio of IAAs including the BCAAs • Higher BV than other proteins • Raises glutathione levels, which stimulates immune system	• Relatively expensive • Needs a blender to mix well
Casein	Milk	• Slower to digest, longer transit through gut, so protein may be asborbed more completely • High glutamine content makes it immune-boosting • 'Anti-catabolic' – i.e. reduces muscle breakdown • Good ratio of IAAs	• Lower BCAA content than whey • Relatively expensive
Soy	Soybeans	• 'Supro' soy isolate has high BCAAs content of glutamine and arginine • Numerous health benefits, including cholesterol lowering and prevention of certain cancers	• Variable quality depending on manufacturing process • Relatively expensive
Milk protein	Skimmed milk	• Good amino acid profile • Low cost	• Unsuitable for those with lactose intolerance • Lower BV than whey or casein

Antioxidant supplements

Antioxidant supplements include beta-carotene, lycopene and other carotenoids, vitamin C, vitamin E, selenium, coenzyme Q10, lipoic acid, conjugated linoleic acid, N-acetyl-cysteine (NAC), proanthocyanidins (found in pine bark and grapeseed extract), curcumin (found in turmeric), the amino acids cysteine and methionine, and catechins (found in green tea).

Try to get as many antioxidants as possible from food. It is not possible to replicate what you get from food in a pill. Food contains hundreds of phytochemicals, all of which have slightly different antioxidant actions. Taking a selected few in the form of a supplement will not give you the best protection.

Taking supplements will not stop you producing free radicals nor enhance your strength and performance.[25] However, they will bolster your body's defences against free radicals. Studies have found that supplementation helps reduce the damage to muscles and other tissues caused by exercise, and reduce post-exercise discomfort, swelling and soreness.[26]

Creatine

Creatine is a protein made naturally in the body from three amino acids (glycine, arginine and methionine). You can also obtain it from fish, beef and pork, although you would need to eat at least 2 kg/day to get a performance-boosting effect. In the muscle cells, it combines with phosphate to make phosphocreatine (PC). PC is an energy-producing compound that regenerates adenosine triphosphate (ATP, a compound that provides energy) extremely rapidly during high-intensity activity. The idea with creatine supplementation is to increase your muscles' PC content. In theory, the more PC you have, the longer you will be able to sustain high-intensity activity.

Creatine supplementation typically raises PC stores in the muscle by around 20 per cent.[27] In terms of performance, most – although not all – studies have found that creatine supplements can increase strength (as measured by the 1RM), allow you to perform more repetitions (at 70 per cent 1RM) before reaching failure, and enable you to recover faster between sets.[28] This would allow you to increase your training volume (i.e. lift heavier weights, perform more repetitions) and therefore lead to greater stimulation for muscle growth.

The original creatine-loading strategy – 20 g/day for five days – used in the studies of the 1990s may lead to excessive water retention. Studies have found that lower doses – 3 g creatine/day for 30 days or 6 g/day (in 6 x 1 g doses) for six days[32] – are just as effective and result in less water retention.

Take creatine with meals or snacks. Protein and carbohydrate stimulate insulin release, which increases creatine uptake by the muscles. Expensive supplements combining creatine with maltodextrin (carbohydrate) or other com-

Creatine and muscle mass

In terms of muscle growth, studies have also found that creatine supplements promote muscle hypertrophy and produce significant gains in total body weight, muscle size and muscle mass.[29] For example, researchers at Pennsylvania State University measured a total body weight gain of 1.7 kg and muscle mass gain of 1.5 kg after seven days of creatine supplementation in a group of 19 weight trainers.[30] After 12 weeks, total weight gain averaged 4.8 kg and muscle mass gain averaged 4.3 kg. Weight gain is partly due to increased cell water content and partly due to increased protein content.[31] Creatine draws water into the muscle cells and this increased cell volume becomes an anabolic signal for muscle growth. Protein breakdown is reduced and protein manufacture increased.

Side effects of creatine

Reports of side effects such as muscle cramps, stomach discomfort, dehydration, and muscle and kidney damage have not been proven. Researchers at the School of Biomedical Sciences at Nottingham University analysed blood samples of volunteers after taking a standard five-day loading dose of creatine followed by a 3 g maintenance dose for nine weeks. They found no evidence of liver, muscle or kidney damage, and concluded that creatine has no health risks in healthy people when taken in the recommended doses.[34] The only 'side effect' appears to be water retention-related weight gain. However, this is associated mainly with the high creatine loading doses (20–30 g/day), and lower loading doses of 6 g/day or less result in very little water retention.

pounds, have not been proven to be more beneficial than plain creatine monohydrate taken with food – and you could end up taking in a lot of unwanted calories.

The ideal amount of carbohydrate is debatable. Studies at Creighton University in Omaha, Nebraska, have found 34 g carbohydrate to be just as effective as the higher doses (80–100 g) used in previous research.[33] Drink extra water when loading with creatine to compensate for the increased uptake of water by your muscle cells.

HMB (beta-hydroxy beta-methylbutyrate)

HMB is a metabolite of the BCAA leucine. Your body breaks down leucine into HMB, but you can also get it from grapefruit, catfish and alfalfa. HMB is a precursor to a component of cell membranes, which helps with the growth and repair of muscle tissue. Its role is not yet clear but scientists believe it either helps protect the muscle from excessive breakdown during intense exercise or accelerates muscle repair after training.

Studies at Iowa State University have suggested that HMB increases muscle mass and strength, and reduces body fat levels, although the exact mechanism is not clear.[35,36] However, researchers at the Australian Institute of Sport found no such effects.[37] Also it appears to have no effect in experienced weight trainers.[38]

Glutamine

Glutamine is a non-essential amino acid that makes up 5–7 per cent of muscle protein. It can be broken down to supply energy during intense training. Glutamine also fuels your immune system.

It has been suggested that glutamine supplements help preserve muscle mass and bolster your immune system during periods of intense training. Studies at Oxford University found that taking glutamine supplements immediately after hard training reduced the risk of upper respiratory tract infection.[39] However, there is no evidence that glutamine increases strength, muscle size or performance.

Many brands of meal-replacement products and protein supplements contain glutamine, making a separate supplementation unnecessary.

Prohormone supplements

Prohormone supplements, such as androstenedione and androstenediol, are precursors to testosterone. They are produced in the body but do very little in the way of muscle-building activity themselves. The theory is that prohormone supplements will be converted into testosterone in your body. Testosterone is a powerful anabolic hormone that increases strength, muscle mass and athletic performance.

Despite claims made by the manufacturers, prohormone supplements do not enhance strength, muscle mass or athletic performance when taken in the dosages recommended by the

The effects of prohormones

In the 'Andro Project', researchers at East Tennessee State University carried out a major study of the effects of 'andro' supplements in 50 men aged 35–65, and found no evidence to back up the manufacturers' claims.[41] The men took part in a 12-week weight training programme and were given either 200 mg androstenedione, 200 mg androstenediol or a placebo (dummy pill). Although testosterone levels increased by 16 per cent after one month in those taking the androstenedione, by the end of 12 weeks they went back to normal. That's because their bodies shut down their own production of testosterone. All the men got stronger during the 12-week programme but there was no difference between those taking the 'andro' supplements and those taking the placebo. What's more, levels of the female hormone oestrogen rose in those using supplements! This could lead to feminisation over a period of time, the opposite of what male strength trainers want to achieve.

manufacturers. Relatively high doses (300 mg), may raise testosterone levels, but they still fail to increase strength or muscle mass.[40]

Supplements raise levels of female sex hormones, including oestrogen and its related compounds. This could lead to gynecomastia (breast development) and lowered libido in men. Some manufacturers recommend taking an oestrogen blocker, chrysin, to counteract this side effect. However, there is no evidence that it works. Another serious side effect of 'andro' use is lowered levels of high-density lipoprotein or the 'good' cholesterol, increasing the risk of heart disease.

Two more good reasons not to take these supplements are the danger of contamination and the risk of failing a drugs test. In a study carried out at the University of California, Los Angeles, all those taking androstenedione were found to have high levels of 19-norandrosterone (the standard marker for nandrolone use) in their urine.[42] The levels were high enough to 'test positive' in a drugs test for steroids. 'Andro' itself does not produce 19-norandrosterone, so researchers concluded that the 'andro' supplements were contaminated with it. When researchers then analysed seven brands of androstenedione, they found that five did not contain the amount stated on the label while one actually contained testosterone!

Most athletic associations, including the International Olympic Committee, ban prohormones, although it is still legal to buy them and they are readily available from manufacturers of nutritional supplements.

Conjugated linoleic acid

Conjugated linoleic acid (CLA) is the collective term for a number of variants of linoleic acid, one of the essential fatty acids (see p. 21). The average diet provides around 100–300 mg CLA/day, mainly from full-fat milk, meat and

Table 3.11	The CLA content of various foods[49]	
Food	Portion	CLA (mg per portion)
Butter	1 tsp (7 g)	76
Yoghurt	1 carton (150 g)	1050
Processed cheese	1 slice (28 g)	169
Cheese	1 slice (28 g)	108
T-bone steak (cooked)	1 small (100 g)	730
Vegetable oil	1 tsp (5 g)	1

The muscle-building benefits of CLA

Research conducted in Norway found that those taking 3,000 mg CLA daily for three months reduced their body fat by 20 per cent.[43] When CLA is combined with strength training, it can reduce muscle breakdown, enhance muscle growth and increase strength. University of Memphis researchers gave 27 experienced weight trainers either 5.6 g CLA/day or an olive oil placebo, and found that CLA improved their strength in the bench press and leg press by 13.6 kg compared with the placebo group's 4.3 kg.[44] Kent State University researchers gave 24 novice bodybuilders either 7.2 g CLA/day or a placebo vegetable oil.[45,46] After six weeks of training the CLA weight trainers had greater gains in arm size (circumference), total muscle mass and enhanced strength — around twice the gains of the placebo group.

cheese. The CLA content of various foods is shown in Table 3.11. Supplements are made from sunflower and safflower oils.

Research shows that CLA can reduce fat storage and increase fat burning. It does this by increasing the activity of an enzyme called hormone sensitive lipase that releases the fat from fat cells into the blood. At the same time it reduces the activity of another enzyme called lipoprotein lipase, which transports fat into the fat cells. The net result is that more fat is burned as fuel and less fat is stored.

Caffeine

Caffeine is a substance that has a pharmacological (drug-like) effect on the body. It is classed as a drug rather than a nutrient but is still considered a nutritional supplement because it is found in many everyday drinks. The caffeine content of coffee varies between 50 and 100 mg/cup, tea contains 30–60 mg/cup, cola 50 mg/330 ml can and caffeinated 'energy' drinks roughly 100 mg/250 ml can.

It has long been used in sport to mask fatigue and increase endurance. The amount needed to get a performance-enhancing effect varies depending on your individual metabolism but studies have used amounts ranging from 3–15 mg/kg body weight (210–1050 mg for a 70 kg athlete). This is equivalent to about three cups of coffee or three cans of caffeinated energy drink. However, as the sensitivity to caffeine varies, you may need to adjust the exact dose. Exceeding 5 mg/kg body weight will not give you further benefit. Until recently, the use of caffeine in drug-tested sports was banned at levels exceeding 5 mg/ml urine. At the time of going to press, it is part of the World Anti-doping Agency's monitoring programme and is no longer on the list of banned stimulants.

Caffeine supplementation has proved beneficial for many types of exercise: short- and long-duration endurance events, as well as high-intensity activities lasting between 5 and 20 minutes.[47] It also benefits power and strength activities: high-intensity running, cycling, rowing and swimming. Researchers at RMIT University, Australia, found that caffeine improved performance and enhanced power output during 2000 m time trials on a rowing ergometer, a power event lasting approximately 7 minutes.[48]

How caffeine works

There are three main theories to explain caffeine's action on athletic performance.

1. In doses above 5 mg/kg body weight (350 mg for a 70 kg athlete), caffeine increases fat burning during exercise while sparing glycogen. It does this by stimulating adrenaline production, which in turn speeds up the release of fatty acids from fat cells into the blood stream. Therefore, taking caffeine before exercise may encourage the muscles to use more fat and less glycogen, and hence postpone fatigue.
2. Caffeine is a stimulant and has a direct effect on muscle contraction. It does this by stimulating the release of calcium from its storage sites in the muscle cells, enabling calcium to stimulate muscle contraction more effectively. This could increase strength and power output.
3. Caffeine stimulates the central nervous system and therefore works at a psychological level. It may increase concentration, mask your perception of fatigue and increase your motivation to train hard.

Caffeine can make you feel more alert and wide-awake. But excessive amounts can cause restlessness, nervousness, trembling, irritability and cause diarrhoea or even heart palpitations. If you are susceptible to caffeine's side effects, it probably isn't worth taking as you won't get a performance-boosting effect. Caffeine is also a diuretic, causing you to excrete more fluid. There is no firm evidence that it causes dehydration, but if you do decide to use caffeine, drink extra water as a precaution before and during exercise to counteract the diuretic effect.

SUMMARY OF KEY POINTS

- To gain weight, you need to take in more calories (approximately 120 per cent) than you burn.

- To reduce body fat and maintain muscle, reduce calories by no more than 15 per cent.
- The general guideline for carbohydrate intake is 5–7 g/kg body weight/day.
- It is recommended that strength trainers consume 1.4–1.8 g protein/kg body weight/day.
- Fat should contribute 15–30 per cent of calories, with an emphasis on unsaturated fats, and omega-3 fatty acids in particular.
- Eating a low GI meal 2–4 hours before training can help maintain blood sugar levels during your workout.
- Eating five or six times a day, avoiding large gaps between meals, promotes efficient recovery between workouts, stimulates the metabolism and reduces the chances of fat gain.
- Carbohydrate plus protein, in a ratio of approximately 3:1, promotes the fastest post-exercise recovery of glycogen and creates a more favourable anabolic environment for muscle growth.

- Aim to consume at least 1.5–2 litres fluid/day plus an additional 150–350 ml every 15–20 minutes during training. Water is the best choice for workouts lasting less than one hour; sports drinks containing carbohydrate are beneficial for longer workouts.
- Vitamin and mineral needs are likely to be higher than those of the general population and the published RDAs – a multivitamin and mineral supplement can act as a good insurance policy.
- Taking extra antioxidants may be helpful in reducing free radical damage caused by exercise.
- Most – though not all – studies suggest creatine supplements help increase body weight, muscle mass, strength and total training volume.
- There is not enough convincing evidence to support the claims for HMB, glutamine or prohormone supplements.

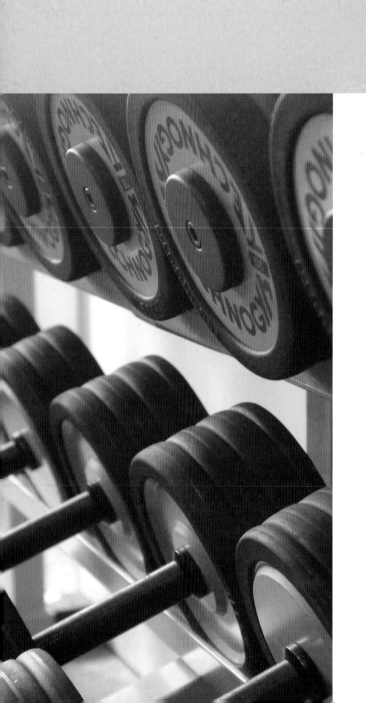

PART **TWO**

THE EXERCISES

In the following chapters, you'll learn how to execute more than 100 exercises with perfect technique. The exercises are divided up by body part: lower body, back, chest, shoulders, arms and abdominals. Each exercise includes step-by-step instructions, technique tips and extra pointers on how to make the exercise harder or easier. There are two photographs demonstrating each exercise, one at the start position and one at the mid-point position. Use these photographs as a guide to correct technique but, in case of doubt, seek the advice of a qualified instructor.

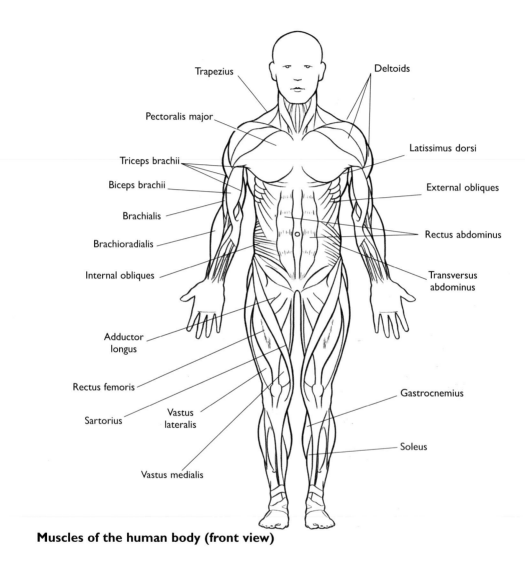

Trapezius

Deltoids

Pectoralis major

Latissimus dorsi

Triceps brachii

Biceps brachii

External obliques

Brachialis

Brachioradialis

Rectus abdominus

Internal obliques

Transversus
abdominus

Adductor
longus

Rectus femoris

Gastrocnemius

Vastus
lateralis

Sartorius

Soleus

Vastus medialis

Muscles of the human body (front view)

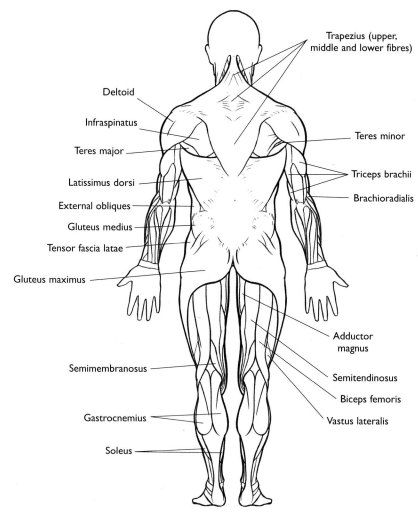

Trapezius (upper, middle and lower fibres)

Deltoid

Infraspinatus

Teres major

Latissimus dorsi

External obliques

Gluteus medius

Tensor fascia latae

Gluteus maximus

Teres minor

Triceps brachii

Brachioradialis

Adductor magnus

Semimembranosus

Semitendinosus

Biceps femoris

Vastus lateralis

Gastrocnemius

Soleus

Muscles of the human body (back view)

THE LOWER BODY

4

Strong, powerful legs give your body good symmetry, balancing the development of the upper body, and facilitating good performance in other sports.

Building a good foundation of strength in the lower body is important in all sports that require running, jumping, lifting, kicking and pushing. Hip and leg extension play a major role in:

- running – as seen in athletics, football and rugby
- jumping – as seen in volleyball and netball
- kicking – as seen in football and the martial arts.

Lower body exercises not only build strength in the hips and thighs but also stimulate muscle growth in the upper body.[1] This is because intense leg training (with weights equivalent to 3–6 RM) stimulates the release of anabolic hormones – namely testosterone and growth hormone – which, in turn, improve whole-body muscle growth.

Training the legs with high intensity will also elevate your heart rate and this, together with the resulting muscle mass increase, will allow you to burn fat more efficiently.

EXERCISES FOR THE LOWER BODY

Squat
Machine squat
Exercise ball squat
Split squat
Dead lift
Leg press
Leg extension
Front lunge
Reverse lunge
Dumbbell step-ups
Seated leg curl
Straight-leg dead lift
Standing calf raise
One-legged dumbbell calf raise
Calf (or toe) press
Seated calf raise

MUSCLE KNOW-HOW

The leg muscles

There are four parts (heads) to the muscle at the front of the thigh, known as the quadriceps – the rectus femoris, vastus lateralis, vastus medialis and vastus intermedius – whose collective function is to extend (straighten) the knee. The rectus femoris also flexes the hip – i.e. lifts the thigh up and forwards.

The vastus medialis runs along the inside of the thigh to the rectus femoris and can be seen on the inside of the knee when the leg is locked out; the vastus lateralis runs down the outside of the thigh and can be seen on the outside of the knee; the rectus femoris can be seen when the leg is lifted up and forwards slightly; the vastus intermedius cannot readily be seen as it lies underneath the other muscles.

The main inner-thigh muscles are comprised of three adductor muscles – adductor brevis, adductor longus and adductor magnus – whose function is to adduct, or pull, the legs together, while the muscles of the outer thigh – the gluteus minimus and gluteus medius – pull the legs out sideways. The muscles at the back of the leg – the hamstrings – include the biceps femoris (long and short heads), semitendinosus and semimembranosus. They have two main actions: to flex (bend) the knee and also extend the hip (pull the thigh backwards).

The calves are comprised of two muscles: the gastrocnemius and soleus. The gastrocnemius is the larger of the two and lies on top of the soleus. It is worked when the leg is fully straight, and has two distinct lobes, which are visible from behind when the calf is flexed. Its role is to straighten the ankle (plantar flexion), to point the toes, and it also helps bend the knee. The soleus is a broad, flat muscle, which is located beneath the gastrocnemius and also helps straighten the ankle. It sweeps out to the sides and over across the shins, and is worked when the knee is bent at about 90 degrees.

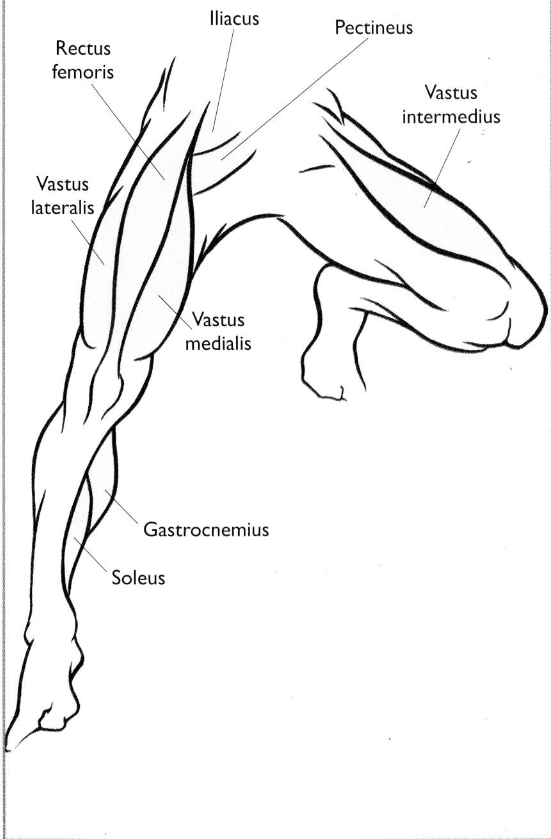

The gluteal muscles

There are three separate muscle groups around the backside, collectively known as the gluteals: gluteus maximus, gluteus medius and gluteus minimus.

Gluteus maximus is the largest, strongest muscle and is largely responsible for the size and shape of the backside. It attaches to the lower vertebrae and top of the rear part of the pelvis, and inserts into the top third of the back of the femur (thigh bone). Its function is to extend the hip in movements such as squatting, stair climbing and rear leg raises.

Gluteus medius is a smaller muscle, attaching at the top of the rear part of the pelvis and inserting at the top of the femur. Its function is to abduct the hip (move the legs out sideways) and also rotate the hip inwards, so it is used on the leg abductor machine or when doing leg raises to the side.

Gluteus minimus is the smallest of the three gluteals, attaching just below the gluteus medius and inserting at the top of the femur. It tends to act as a stabilising muscle, working eccentrically during impact movements such as running and jumping, and holding the hip joint in position.

Figure 4.1 Muscles of the leg

Rectus femoris
Iliacus
Pectineus
Vastus intermedius
Vastus lateralis
Vastus medialis
Gastrocnemius
Soleus

Figure 4.2 The gluteal muscles

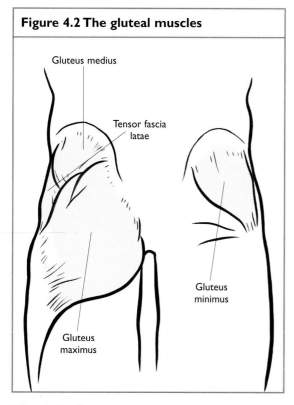

Figure 4.3 The hip flexors

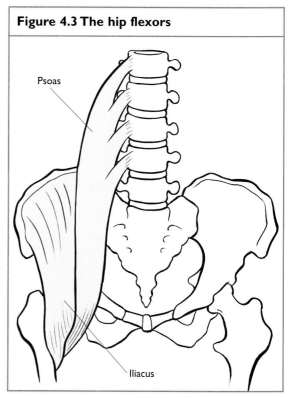

The hip flexors

The main hip flexors are the iliacus, psoas (ilop-soas), rectus femoris, pectineus and tensor fascia latae. The iliacus and psoas muscles cannot be seen as they lie deep in the abdomen, running from the lower vertebrae to the top of the thigh bone. They flex the hip. The psoas muscles also help to stabilise the lower back. One of the quadriceps group of muscles, the rectus femoris, runs down the front of the thigh and crosses both the hip joint and the knee joint. It flexes the hip as well as the knee. The pectineus is a short muscle located close to the groin. It is partly covered by the rectus femoris. The tensor fascia latae can be seen on the outer front part of the hip. It helps to flex the hips as well as move the leg outwards.

SQUAT

Target muscles

Gluteals, quadriceps, hamstrings, lower back, adductors, hip flexors

The squat is one of the most efficient exercises for increasing mass, strength and power in the lower body. It is a compound movement that involves many stabiliser muscles to complete the lift.

Starting position

1. Position the bar across the upper part of your back so it is resting on your trapezius muscles (not your neck). Alternatively, you may hold a pair of dumbbells by your sides (one at each side).

2. Firmly grip the bar, with your hands almost double shoulder-width apart. As you lift the bar off the rack, ensure there is a normal curve (neutral alignment) in your lower back.

3. Position your feet shoulder-width apart (or slightly wider), toes angled out at 30 degress.

The movement

1. Keeping your head up and your body erect, slowly lower yourself down until your thighs are parallel to the ground; it is not wise to go any further than this. Keep your knees aligned over your feet, pointing in the direction of your toes. Hold for a count of one.

2. From here, press the weight up, pushing hard through your feet and keeping your body erect as you return to the starting position.

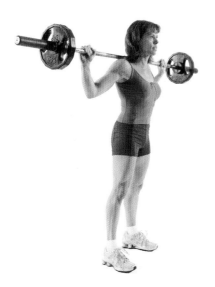
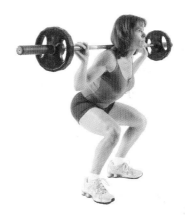

Tips

- You should maintain the natural curve in your back throughout the movement.
- If you lack ankle flexibility, it's better to work on this to improve your ROM rather than to use a board under your heels. This is potentially dangerous for the knees because it moves the knees forwards over the feet and can actually reduce your flexibility.
- Breathe in as you lower the weight, allowing your chest to expand and pulling your tummy button in towards your spine. Exhale as you push upwards.
- Keep your eyes fixed on a point in front of you at about eye level.
- Make sure you do not bend forwards excessively or curve your back as this will stress your lower back and reduce the emphasis on your legs.
- Keep your hips under the bar as much as possible and your knees tracking over your toes as you rise.
- Do not rely on a weight belt unless you are using maximal weight or it could result in a weakening of the abdominal muscles. The abdominal wall should be drawn in towards the spine rather than pushing out against a belt when lifting.

Variations

WIDER STANCE

Placing your feet just over shoulder-width apart (but not too far or you may lose stability) and taking the squat slightly deeper than parallel places more emphasis on the gluteals on the upward part of the movement. Make sure you practise perfect form and control the squat – you will have to reduce the weight on the bar, since going deeper can put greater strain on the knees. You'll find this technique will not only increase your overall strength but will also shape your gluteals!

SMITH MACHINE SQUATS

Squats performed using a Smith machine are less effective than barbell squats and may increase injury risk when you are not using a machine as it does not develop the stabiliser muscles. Since the bar travels in a straight line, this alters your natural movement, taking much of the emphasis away from your all-important stabilising muscles. If you must use a Smith machine, position your feet so that your heels are directly under the bar.

MACHINE SQUAT

Target muscles

Gluteals, quadriceps, hamstrings, lower back, adductors, hip flexors

Squats performed on an angled machine are comparable to free weight squats except that you don't have to balance a bar, just push against the resistance through your shoulders. This makes it somewhat easier and reduces the chances of injury.

Starting position

1. Position your shoulders under the pads of the machine.
2. Place your feet hip-width apart on the platform, your toes pointed directly in front of you and (depending on the machine) your feet out slightly in front of your body.

The movement

1. Release the safety mechanism of the machine and slowly lower the weight under control.
2. Lower your body until your thighs are parallel with the floor (approximately 90 degrees between your thigh and lower leg), while maintaining the normal arch in your spine.
3. From here, reverse directions and rise, pushing hard through your feet as you return to the starting position.

Tips

• Maintain the natural curve in your back throughout the movement.
• Your knees should remain directly over your feet at all times.
• Breathe in as you lower the weight and breathe out as you push upwards.

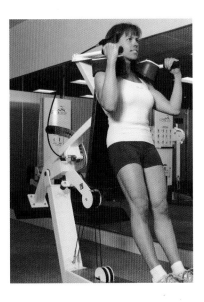
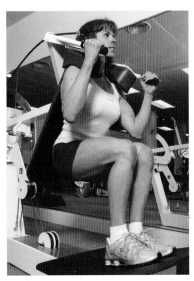

EXERCISE BALL SQUAT

Target muscles

Gluteals, quadriceps, hamstrings

Starting position

1. Put an exercise ball just behind you against a wall. Stand with your lower back firmly against it.
2. Position your feet shoulder-width apart slightly further forwards than your shoulders. Cross you arms over your chest.

The movement

1. Slowly bend your knees to roll the ball down the wall. Lower until your thighs are parallel to the ground, maintaining the normal arch in your spine.
2. Pressing through your heels, raise yourself back up again as you straighten your legs.

Tips

• Keep the normal curvature in your spine by contracting your abdominals.
• Look directly ahead.

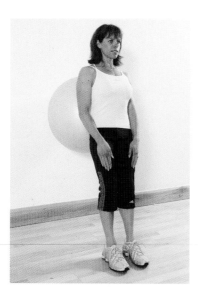
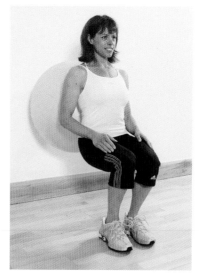

SPLIT SQUAT

Target muscles

Gluteals, hamstrings, quadriceps

Starting position

1. Position the bar of a Smith machine across the upper part of your back so it is resting on your trapezius muscles (not your neck). Alternatively, hold a pair of dumbbells at your sides (one at each side) with your palms facing your body.
2. Take a step forwards with your right leg and a step back with your left. Your left heel will lift off the floor. The bar should be midway between your two feet.

The movement

1. Drop your body downwards, bending your right knee to 90 degrees, bringing your rear knee to a point just above the floor.
2. Push through the front heel to press back up into a standing split squat.
3. Complete the desired repetitions for one side, and then switch legs to complete the set.

Tips

- When descending, think about dropping your hips straight down so you avoid bending forwards.
- Keep your head level, chest out and back straight.
- Keep your front knee positioned directly over your ankle – do not allow it to extend further forwards.

Variation

ON A BLOCK

Put your rear foot on a block or step about 15 cm high. This increases the range of motion and you will feel a greater stretch in the quadriceps of the rear leg.

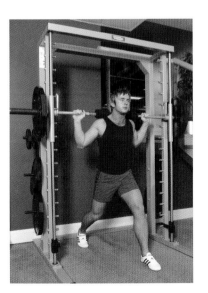
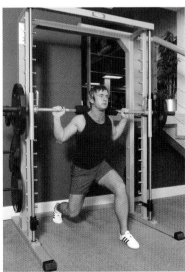

DEAD LIFT

Target muscles

Gluteus maximus, quadriceps, hamstrings, hip flexors, lower back, adductors, latissimus dorsi, trapezius, abdominals

The dead lift is a fundamental exercise for increasing overall mass, strength and power in both the lower and upper body. Like squats, it is a maximum-stimulation movement.

Starting position

1. Stand in front of the barbell with your feet parallel and shoulder-width apart.
2. Bend your legs until your hips and knees are at the same level, keeping your rib cage up and your head level. Your back should be straight, at a 45-degree angle to the floor.
3. Grasp the bar, with your hands just over shoulder-width apart, one overhand, the other under. This will facilitate better balance and keep the barbell in the same plane.

The movement

1. Using the power of your legs and hips, and keeping your arms straight, lift the bar from the floor until your legs are straight. The bar should rest against the upper part of your thighs. Hold for a count of one.
2. Slowly return the bar to the floor, keeping your torso erect, arms straight and head up, eyes looking forwards. Your chest should be slightly forwards and over the bar.

Tips

- Maintain the normal curvature of your spine throughout the movement – do not lean forwards or tilt backwards.
- Keep your abdominals and lower back muscles contracted to support your spine.
- Drive the movement from your hip muscles – make sure you don't pull with the arms.
- Keep the bar as close as possible to your legs throughout the movement.
- Make sure your knees travel in line with your toes – do not allow them to travel inwards.

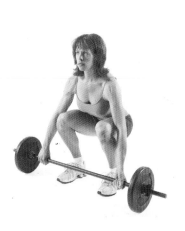

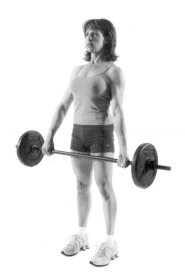

LEG PRESS

Target muscles

Gluteals, quadriceps, hamstrings

Also a good strength and mass builder for the lower body, the leg press is often preferred by those with weak lower-back muscles. There is little involvement of the stabiliser muscles and this, paradoxically, may lead to further weakening or imbalance of the deep muscles close to the spine and pelvis. To reduce injury risk, keep your lower back flat on the support.

Starting position

1. Sit into the base of the leg press machine (seated, lying or incline) with your back firmly against the padding.
2. Position your feet parallel and hip-width apart on the platform.
3. Release the safety bars and extend your legs.

The movement

1. Slowly bend your legs and lower the platform in a controlled fashion until your knees almost touch your chest. Hold for a count of one.
2. Return the platform to the starting position, pushing hard through your heels.

Tips

- Keep your back in full contact with the base; do not allow your lower spine to curl up as you lower the platform.
- Keep your knees in line with your toes.
- Do not 'snap out' or lock your knees as you straighten your legs back to the starting position.
- Make sure you do not bounce your knees off your chest.

Variations

WIDE FOOT SPACING

Placing your feet shoulder-width apart with your toes angled outwards puts more emphasis on the inner thigh muscles and will therefore help to develop this part of the thigh.

FEET HIGHER ON PLATFORM

Placing your feet higher on the platform so that your toes are almost off the edge puts more emphasis on the hamstrings and gluteals, and will therefore help develop these muscles.

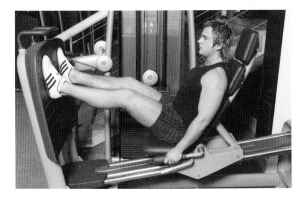
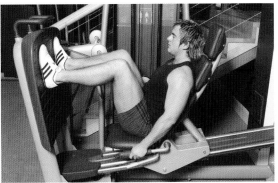

LEG EXTENSION

Target muscles

Quadriceps

This exercise helps to develop the front thigh muscles, particularly the 'teardrop' muscles that hold the knee.

Starting position

1. Sit on the leg extension machine, adjusting it so that the back of your thighs are fully supported on the seat.
2. Hook your feet under the foot pads. The pads should rest on the lowest part of your shins, just above your ankles.
3. Hold on to the sides of the seat or the handles on the sides of the machine to prevent your hips lifting as you perform the exercise.

The movement

1. Straighten your legs to full extension, keeping your thighs and backside fully in contact with the bench.
2. Hold this fully contracted position for a count of two, then slowly return to the starting point.

Tips

- Do not allow your hips to raise off the seat.
- Try to 'resist' the weight as you lower your legs back to the starting point – avoid letting the weight swing your legs back.
- Make sure you fully straighten the leg until the knees are locked – do not perform partial movements.
- Avoid swinging/kicking your legs – control the movement.

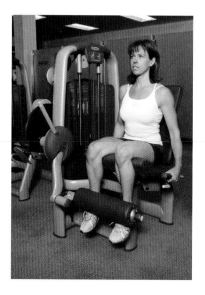
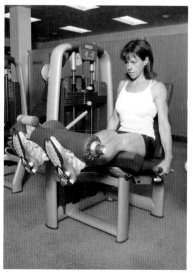

FRONT LUNGE (DUMBBELL OR BARBELL)

Target muscles

Quadriceps, hamstrings, gluteals

Starting position

1. Hold a pair of dumbbells at the sides of your body with arms fully extended (palms facing your body) or place a bar across the back of your shoulders.
2. Stand with your feet shoulder-width apart, toes pointing forwards. Look straight ahead.

The movement

1. Take an exaggerated step forwards with your right leg, bending the knee and lowering your hips.
2. Lower yourself until your right thigh is parallel to the floor and your knee is at an angle of 90 degrees. Your left leg should be about 10–15 cm above the floor. Hold for a count of one.
3. Push hard with your right leg to return to the starting position.
4. Complete the desired number of repetitions, then repeat with the left leg leading.

Tips

• Keep your front knee positioned directly over your ankle – do not allow it to extend further forwards as this can cause strain to the knee.
• Keep your body erect throughout the movement – do not lean forwards.

Variations

STEP LENGTH

A shorter step forwards places more emphasis on the quadriceps; a larger step forwards places more emphasis on the gluteal and hamstring muscles.

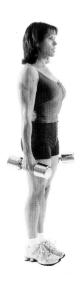

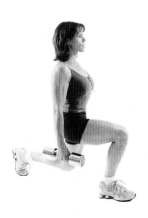

REVERSE LUNGE

Target muscles

Gluteals, hamstrings, quadriceps

Starting position

1. Place a barbell across the back of your shoulders or hold a pair of dumbbells at the sides of your body.
2. Stand with your feet shoulder-width apart, toes pointing forwards.

The movement

1. Drop your right leg behind your body, bending your left leg, lowering your hips and keeping your trunk upright.
2. Lower yourself into a one-legged squat position on your left leg until your left thigh is parallel to the floor. Your left knee should be at an angle of 90 degrees. Hold for a count of one.
3. Push hard through your left leg, strongly contracting the gluteals, quadriceps and hamstrings to return your right leg into position. Don't push through your right (back) leg.
4. Complete the desired number of repetitions, then repeat with the left leg leading.

Tips

- Keep your front knee positioned directly over your ankle – do not allow it to extend further forwards.
- Keep your body erect and your spine in its neutral position throughout the movement – do not lean forwards and do not round your lower back.
- Make sure you step back far enough so that when you lower your body, the knee of your front leg doesn't pass your toes. In the bottom position your shin should be vertical.

Variation

SMITH MACHINE REVERSE LUNGE

Stand directly under the bar of the Smith machine so that it rests fairly low across your upper back while still allowing you to maintain an upright posture. Hold the bar and lift it from the rack, unlocking the safety catches. Perform the movement as above.

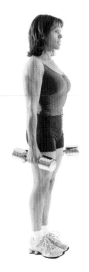

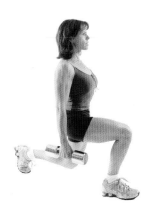

DUMBBELL STEP-UPS

Starting position

1. Stand holding a pair of dumbbells facing a step that is approximately 30–45 cm high.

> ### Target muscles
> Quadriceps, gluteals, hamstrings

The movement

1. Step up on to the step with one leg then lift your other foot on top of the step.

2. Step down with the second leg then the first.
3. Repeat with the second leg leading.

Tips

- Do not allow your body to lean forwards while stepping up.
- Make sure your foot is securely on top of the step when you step up.
- Increase the height of the step to work your muscles harder.

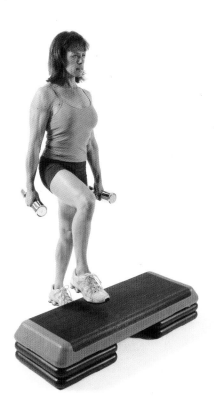
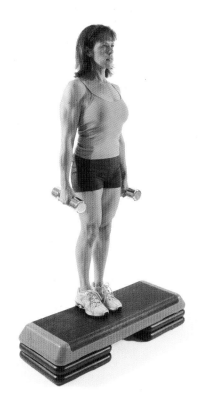

SEATED LEG CURL

Target muscles

Hamstrings
Also used: gastrocnemius

Starting position

1. Sit down in the leg curl machine and place your heels over the roller pads. Adjust the machine if necessary so that your knees are just off the end of the bench and your thighs fully supported.

2. Hold on to the hand grips or the edge of the bench for support.

The movement

1. Bend your knees, bringing your heels towards your backside.
2. Hold this fully contracted position for a count of two then slowly lower your heels back to the starting position.

Tips

• Control the movement on both the upwards and downwards phase; avoid kicking your heels back fast.

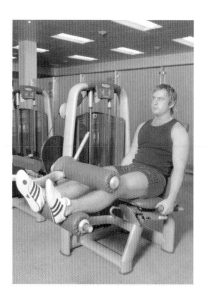
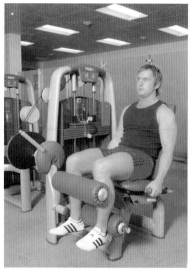

STRAIGHT-LEG DEAD LIFT

Target muscles

Hamstrings, gluteals, lower back

This exercise requires a high degree of technical skill and flexibility so is unsuitable for beginners and anyone with lower back problems. Performed correctly, it can work the hamstrings even more effectively than the leg curl.

Starting position

1. Grasp a barbell with your hands slightly wider than shoulder-width apart, using an overhand grip.
2. Stand up straight, looking directly ahead.

The movement

1. Keep your back flat and legs nearly straight.
2. Bend forwards from the hips until your back is parallel to the ground. You should feel a stretch in your hamstrings and gluteals. As you bend forwards, your hips and gluteals should move backwards and your body should be centred through your heels.
3. At the bottom of the movement, do not allow the weight to touch the floor and don't round your back.
4. Hold for a count of one then forcefully contract your gluteals and hamstrings to raise your torso back into the erect starting position.

Tips

- Keep your back flat. Rounding your back will increase the risk of injury.
- Do not lower the bar too far. The bar should be hanging at arm's length below you, at about knee level. Going below this point hyperflexes the spine, putting it in a vulnerable position and increasing injury risk to the lower back.
- Concentrate on using your hips as a hinge.

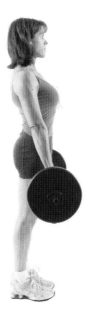
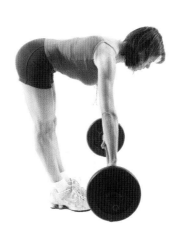

STANDING CALF RAISE

Target muscles

Gastrocnemius, soleus

This is perhaps the best exercise for overall development of the calves.

Starting position

1. Place your shoulders under the pads of a standing calf raise machine or Smith machine. Alternatively, place a barbell across the back of your shoulders, resting on your trapezius muscles (not your neck).
2. Step on to the platform or, if you are using a barbell, use a step or block. Allow your heels to hang off the edge.
3. Stand with your feet hip-width apart and pointing directly ahead.
4. Straighten your legs as you lift the selected weight clear of the rest of the stack.

The movement

1. Rise up on your toes as high as possible.
2. Hold the fully contracted position for a count of two, then slowly lower your heels as far as they will go.

Tips

- Keep your legs straight (but not locked) throughout the movement to keep maximal emphasis on the calves and reduce the involvement of the quadriceps.
- Maintain a tight, naturally vertical plane, keeping the natural arch in your back, and your head and neck in a neutral position.
- Stretch your calves fully at the bottom of the movement – your heels should be lower than your toes.
- Do not bounce up from the bottom – keep the movement smooth and continuous.

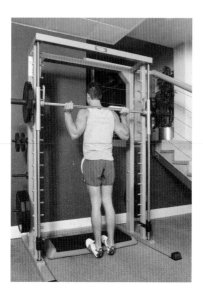
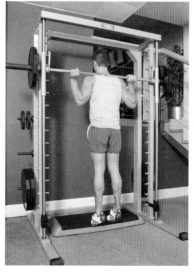

ONE-LEGGED DUMBBELL CALF RAISE

Target muscles

Gastrocnemius, soleus

This exercise is similar to that on a standing calf raise machine but is done one leg at a time.

Starting position

1. Hold a dumbbell in your right hand with your arm hanging down by your side, palm facing your body.
2. Place the ball of the right foot on the edge of a block or platform, allowing your heel to hang off the edge.
3. Hold on to a suitable support with the other hand to steady yourself.

The movement

1. Rise up as high as possible on the ball of your foot.
2. Hold the fully contracted position for a count of two, then slowly lower your heel as far as it will go.
3. Complete the desired number of repetitions, then repeat on the left leg.

Tips

- Keep your exercising leg straight throughout the movement.
- Keep your body upright.
- Stretch your calf fully at the bottom of the movement – your heel should be lower than your toes.
- Keep the movement smooth and continuous.

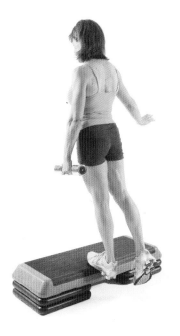 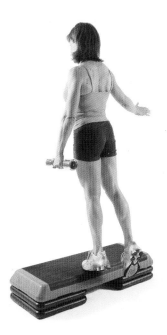

CALF (OR TOE) PRESS

Target muscles

Gastrocnemius, soleus

Starting position

1. Position yourself in a leg press machine.
2. Place the balls of your feet on the bottom of the platform with your heels hanging off the edge. Your legs should be fully extended and feet hip-width apart. Release the safety catch.

The movement

1. Press the platform away from you as far as possible.
2. Hold the fully contracted position for a count of two, then slowly lower your heels as far as they will go.

Tips

- Stretch your calves fully at the bottom of the movement.
- Keep your legs straight (not locked) throughout the movement.

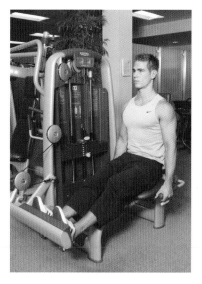
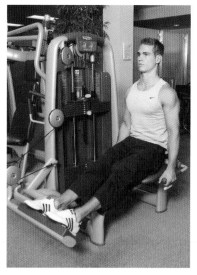

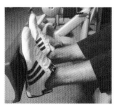
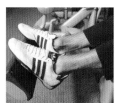

SEATED CALF RAISE

Target muscles

Soleus

Starting position

1. Sit on a bench in front of a step and place a barbell across your lower thighs.
   Alternatively, position yourself on a seated calf raise machine, adjusting the pad height to fit snugly over your lower thighs.
2. Place the balls of your feet on the step, making sure they are directly below your knees.

The movement

1. Rise up on to the balls of your feet and hold for a moment.
2. Then slowly lower your heels until they are as far below the balls of your feet as possible.
3. Complete the desired number of repetitions.

Tips

- Make sure you move through a full range of movement.
- To maximally stress the soleus muscle, hold the uppermost position for at least two seconds.

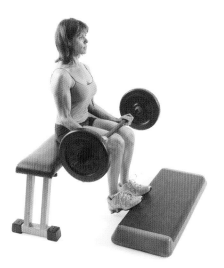
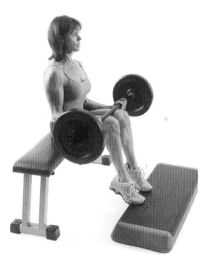

THE BACK

5

Training your back will change the proportions of your entire body. Well-developed latissimus dorsi muscles (lats) create that classic V-shape, making your waist appear smaller and, for women, balancing the curves of the lower body.

Strong back muscles are important in sports that involve pulling actions, such as rowing. These actions are used in rugby tackling, judo, boxing, gymnastics and swimming, especially butterfly and front crawl. A strong back will also help you develop other major muscle groups, as your back assists in key exercises such as squatting, shoulder presses and standing biceps curls; while having a strong back helps in everyday activities, such as lifting and carrying, and prevents back injuries.

EXERCISES FOR THE UPPER BACK

Lat pull-down
Pull-up/chin-up
One-arm dumbbell row
Seated cable row
Bent-over barbell row
Straight-arm pull-downs
Machine row
Dumbbell pull-over
Dumbbell shrug

EXERCISES FOR THE LOWER BACK

Back extension (on the floor)
Dorsal raise
Back extension with exercise ball

MUSCLE KNOW-HOW

The major muscles in the upper back include: the trapezius, the diamond-shaped muscle which extends from the back of the neck to the mid-back (this may be divided into upper and mid-portions) and which draws the shoulder blades backwards and upwards – as well as turning the head and bending it backwards; the latissimus dorsi ('lats'), the large wing-like muscles running from your shoulders to your waist that make up the majority of the muscle mass of the upper and mid-back, and which draw the arms downwards; the rhomboids (lying beneath the mid-part of the trapezius in the central upper back), which help draw the shoulder blades backwards; and the smaller infraspinatus, supraspinatus, teres major and teres minor muscles, which are located around the shoulder blades and rotate the arms outwards.

The erector spinae running along the sides of the mid- and lower spine straighten the trunk from a flexed position, as well as moving the trunk sideways. They work in concert with the abdominals and oblique muscles to stabilise the torso (see p. 109).

Figure 5.1 Muscles of the back

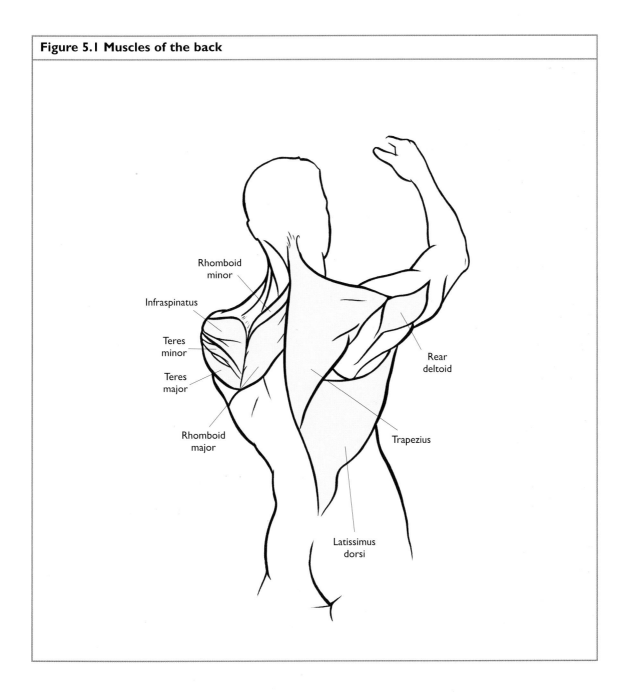

LAT PULL-DOWN

Target muscles

Latissimus dorsi, rhomboids
Also used: biceps, posterior deltoids, forearms

Starting position

1. Hold the bar, with your hands just over shoulder-width apart and palms facing forwards.
2. Sit on the seat, adjusting it so that your knees fit snugly under the roller pads. Your arms should be fully extended.

The movement

1. Pull the bar down towards your chest until it touches the upper part of your chest, arching your back slightly.
2. Hold for a count of two, then slowly return to the starting position.

Tips

- Keep your trunk as still as possible.
- Focus on keeping your elbows directly under the bar and squeezing your shoulder blades together.

- Do not shorten the return phase of the movement – extend your arms fully.
- Do not lean back too far.

Variations

CLOSE GRIP

This variation works the inner portion of the latissimus dorsi, thus creating more depth to the mid-back. Use a triangle bar attachment and bring it down in front of your neck until it just touches the mid-point of your chest.

REVERSE GRIP

This variation also thickens the latissimus dorsi rather than widening them, thus creating more depth to the mid-back. Use a short, straight bar attachment and hold the bar with your palms facing you, about 15–20 cm apart.

Behind neck pull-downs

The front pull-down is considered a better exercise than behind neck pull-downs; researchers at the University of Miami found that it produces a more powerful contraction in the muscles. In addition, pulling the bar down behind the neck increases the potential for injury to the shoulder joint and the upper spine. For this reason, you should pull the bar to your chest, not behind your neck.

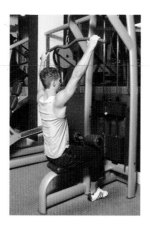
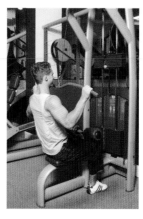

PULL-UP/CHIN-UP

Target muscles

Latissimus dorsi, trapezius, rhomboids, infraspinatus, teres major and minor
Also used: biceps, posterior deltoids, forearms

Starting position

1. Hold the bar with your hands just over shoulder-width apart, palms facing forwards.
2. Your arms should be fully extended and your ankles crossed to prevent your body from swinging around. If you are using a pull-up machine, simply place your feet on the platform.

The movement

1. Pull yourself up slowly until your eyes are level with the bar. Lead with your upper chest.

2. Pause for a second or two, then slowly lower back to the starting position.

Tips

- Do not swing your legs forwards or jerk as you pull yourself up – this greatly reduces the stress placed on the back muscles.
- Fix your eyes slightly upwards as you pull yourself up, arching your back just a little.
- Ensure your trunk and thighs maintain a straight line.
- Do not shorten the return phase of the movement – extend your arms fully.

Variations

CLOSE GRIP

This variation places more stress on the lower lats and biceps. Use either an overhand or underhand grip, with your hands shoulder-width apart.

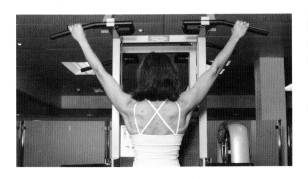

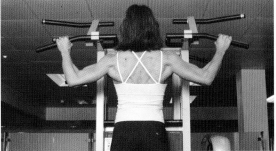

ONE-ARM DUMBBELL ROW

Target muscles

Latissimus dorsi, trapezius, rhomboids, infraspinatus, teres major and minor
Also used: biceps, posterior deltoids

Starting position

1. Hold a dumbbell in your right hand, palm facing your body.
2. Bend forwards from the hips, placing your left hand and knee on a bench to stabilise yourself. Your back should be flat and almost horizontal, and your right arm fully extended.

The movement

1. Pull the dumbbell up towards your waist, drawing your elbow back as far as it can go. Keep the dumbbell close to your body.
2. Allow the dumbbell to touch your rib cage lightly. Pause for a count of one, then lower the dumbbell slowly until your arm is fully extended.
3. After completing the required number of repetitions, perform the exercise with your left arm.

Tips

- Keep your lower back flat and still – do not twist your trunk.
- Make sure you row the dumbbell to the side of your rib cage – do not pull it up to your shoulder.

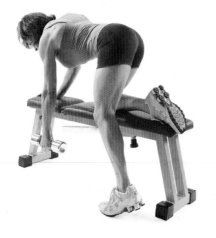 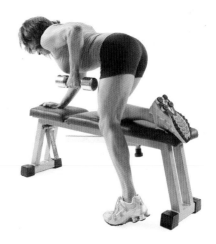

SEATED CABLE ROW

Target muscles

Latissimus dorsi, trapezius, rhomboids, teres major and minor
Also used: erector spinae, biceps, forearms, pectoralis major

Starting position

1. Sit facing the cable row machine and place your feet against the footrests. Grasp the bar and bend your knees slightly.
2. Lean forwards and grasp the pulley handles, while maintaining a normal, slightly curved spinal position.
3. Pull back a little way until your torso is nearly upright and your arms extended fully.

The movement

1. Pull the bar towards you until it touches your lower rib/upper abdomen region. You should be pulling your elbows and shoulders directly backwards as far as possible.
2. Hold for a count of two, then return slowly to the starting position, maintaining a near-upright position.

Tips

- To achieve maximum back development, keep your torso nearly upright during the entire movement – it should not move forwards or backwards more than 10 degrees.
- Maintain a normal curve in your back – do not arch your back excessively.
- Keep your legs slightly bent and still throughout the movement.
- Inhale at the start of the movement, then hold your breath during the pulling phase – this helps stabilise your torso. Exhale only towards the end of the movement once your arms are extended.

Variations

STRAIGHT BAR

Cable rows may be performed using a short, straight bar instead of a triangle bar, with a palms-down grip. This emphasises the posterior deltoids, rhomboids and mid-part of the trapezius.

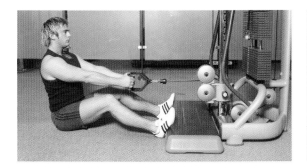

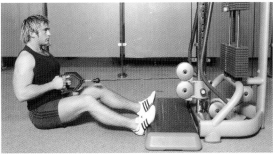

BENT-OVER BARBELL ROW

> **Target muscles**
>
> Latissimus dorsi, trapezius, rhomboids, teres major and minor
> Also used: biceps, forearms

Starting position

1. Place the bar on the floor in front of you.
2. Stand with your feet parallel and shoulder-width apart.
3. Bending forwards from the hips, keeping your back flat and slightly bending your knees, grasp the bar with an overhand grip that is slightly wider than shoulder-width apart.
4. Lift the bar just a short way off the floor. Position your body so that your torso is nearly parallel to the ground, arms fully extended.

The movement

1. Slowly pull the bar towards your lower chest until it just touches the lower part of your rib cage.
2. Hold this position for a count of one, then slowly lower the bar to the starting position.

Tips

- As you pull the bar up, squeeze your shoulder blades together and keep your elbows directly above your hands.
- Keep your back flat throughout the movement – do not round it or you risk injury.
- Keep your torso still – it is tempting to move your torso upwards with the bar to generate momentum. This reduces the work on the back muscles and increases the risk of injury.

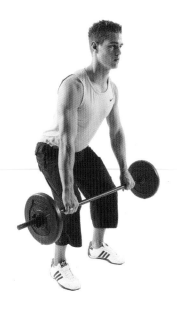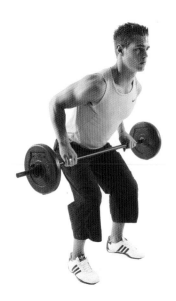

STRAIGHT-ARM PULL-DOWNS

Target muscles

Latissimus dorsi, trapezius, rhomboids, teres major and minor

Starting position

1. Stand in front of a lat pull-down machine.
2. Hold the bar with your arms extended, palms facing downwards.
3. Pull down the bar to shoulder level.

The movement

1. Keeping your arms extended, pull the bar down until it just touches your upper thighs.
2. Hold for a count of two, then slowly return the bar to the starting position.

Tips

- Keep your wrists straight throughout the movement.
- Allow a very slight bend in the elbows – they should not be locked.
- Keep your body still and upright throughout the movement – you will need to use your abdominal muscles to stabilise your torso.

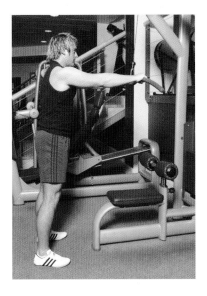 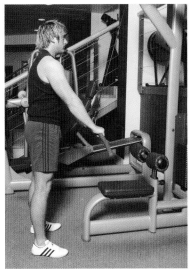

MACHINE ROW

Target muscles

Latissimus dorsi, trapezius, rhomboids, teres major and minor
Also used: biceps, forearms

Starting position

1. Sit with your chest against the support pad and take an overhand grip on the handles.

The movement

1. Pull the handles towards your sides.
2. Hold for a moment then slowly lower the weight and repeat.

Tips

- Maintain the natural curve in your lower back throughout the movement.
- Don't allow the weight stack to touch down between reps.

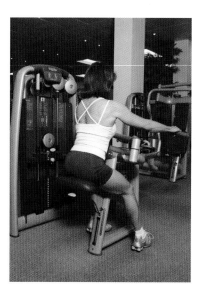
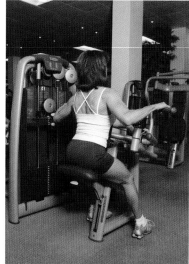

DUMBBELL PULL-OVER

Target muscles

Latissimus dorsi, pectoralis major, triceps

Starting position

1. Lie down perpendicular with just your upper back and shoulders on a flat bench. Your feet should be flat on the floor.
2. Cup your hands around one end of a dumbbell (your palms flat against the top inner plate). Hold the dumbbell over your head with your arms extended.

The movement

1. Slowly lower the dumbbell in a backward arc, down and behind your head, keeping a slight bend in your arms throughout, until your elbows are level with your ears.
2. Raise the dumbbell back over your head using the same arcing motion.

Tips

- Keep your hips lower than your shoulders.
- Avoid arching your back during the movement.
- Don't take the dumbbell back too far – going too deep will increase the risk of shoulder injury.

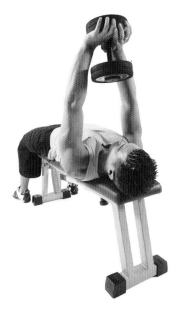
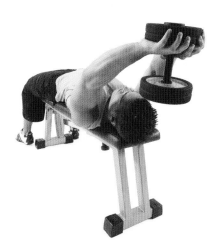

DUMBBELL SHRUG

Target muscles

Trapezius (upper), rhomboids, various other neck and shoulder girdle muscles

Starting position

1. Stand with your feet hip-width apart.
2. Hold a pair of dumbbells by your sides level with your thighs, palms facing backwards. Keep your arms straight.

The movement

1. Raise your shoulders straight up towards your ears, keeping your arms straight.
2. Hold for a count of two, then lower the dumbbells back to the starting position.

Tips

- Keep your arms straight throughout the movement.
- Lift and lower the dumbbells slowly and deliberately – don't jerk them.
- As you lower the dumbbells, allow your shoulders to drop down as far as possible – this stretches the trapezius and increases the ROM.
- Do not rotate your shoulders backwards at the top of the movement – this increases the risk of injury to the shoulder and places no further work on the trapezius.
- Use straps to improve your grip.

Variation

BARBELL SHRUG

Shrugs may be performed with a barbell instead of dumbbells. Hold a barbell in front of or behind your thighs, keep your arms straight and move the bar up and down as described above.

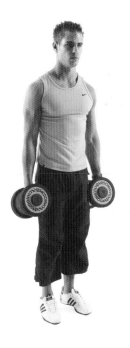
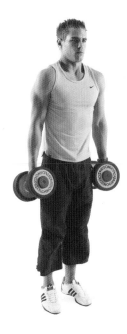

BACK EXTENSION (ON THE FLOOR)

Target muscles

Erector spinae, gluteals

The lower back muscles rarely work through their full ROM during daily activities, nor during exercises for other muscle groups. While the lower back is often involved as a stabiliser in other exercises, such as squats, it is important to include a specific back extension movement in your back workout, which targets the muscles effectively and makes everyday activities easier to perform with less injury risk.

Starting position

1. Lie face down on a mat or the floor.
2. Place your hands by the sides of your head, elbows out to the sides. Alternatively, your arms may be placed behind you, resting on your back.

The movement

1. Slowly raise your head, shoulders and upper chest from the floor. This will be just a short distance.

2. Pause for a count of two, then lower slowly to the floor.

Tips

- Keep your head facing downwards to the floor in line with your spine.
- Keep your legs relaxed on the floor – do not raise them.
- Only raise yourself as far as you feel comfortable.

Variations

BACK EXTENSION BENCH

Tuck your ankles underneath the pads and position your body so that your hips are resting on the middle pad, arms crossed in front of you. Raise your torso until you are parallel with the floor – do not rise higher than this. Slowly bend forwards at the waist until you are almost perpendicular to the floor. Keep your back flat.

To make the movement harder, place your hands along the sides of your head. Alternatively, if you are an advanced weight trainer, hold a small weight disc against your chest.

BACK EXTENSION WITH ROTATION

This exercise targets the spinal rotating muscles. As you lift your upper body off the floor, slowly rotate, turning your shoulders to one side. Return to the central position then lower.

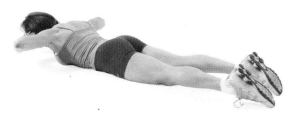
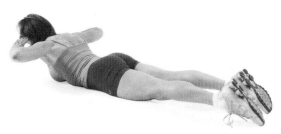

DORSAL RAISE

Target muscles

Erector spinae, gluteals

Starting position

1. Lie face down on a mat with your arms stretched out in front of you and your legs straight.

The movement

1. Slowly raise your left arm and your right leg, keeping them both straight. This will be just a short distance.
2. Hold for a count of two, then lower slowly to the floor. Repeat, raising the opposite arm and leg.

Tips

- Keep your head facing downwards to the floor in line with your spine.
- Only raise as far as you feel comfortable.

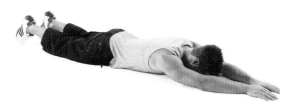

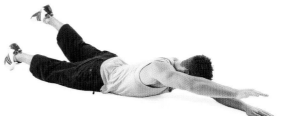

BACK EXTENSION WITH EXERCISE BALL

Target muscles

Erector spinae, gluteals

Starting position

1. Lie over an exercise ball (also called a Swiss ball), face down, keeping your hips halfway up the ball rather than balanced on top of it. Place your feet against a wall for support if you like.
2. Place your arms either crossed over your chest or by the sides of your head.
3. Keep your legs wide and straight out behind you.

The movement

1. Raise your upper body slowly in a straight line towards the ceiling.
2. Hold for a count of two, then lower again slowly.

Tips

- Do not arch your back.
- Keep your head in line with your spine.
- To make the movement harder, bring your legs closer together.

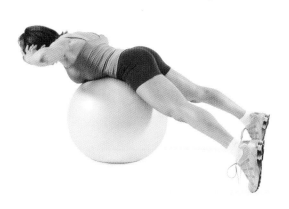
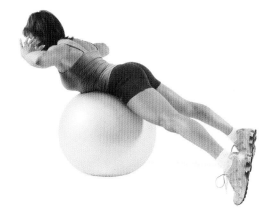

THE CHEST

6

The desire for a bigger, better-developed chest is perhaps the greatest motivator for men to strength train. It somehow symbolises heroism and male virility. Women, too, can benefit from chest training. Although it won't increase the size of your breasts (they are mostly fat tissue), it will create the appearance of a fuller and more shapely chest.

Strong chest muscles are advantageous in many sports. These muscles are involved in all forward- and upward-reaching actions – e.g. in rugby tackling and grabbing an opponent – and are also used in throwing and hitting movements – e.g. during forehand drives in tennis and squash; when throwing the ball overhead in netball, basketball and volleyball; throwing the discus and javelin, and putting the shot. A strong chest is also advantageous in swimming (breaststroke) and several gymnastic disciplines.

EXERCISES FOR THE CHEST

Barbell bench press
Vertical bench press machine
Dumbbell press
Incline barbell bench press
Incline dumbbell bench press
Dumbbell flye
Pec-deck flye
Cable cross-over
Low-pulley cable cross-over
Exercise ball press-up/push-up

MUSCLE KNOW-HOW

The largest muscle of the chest is the pectoralis major, which attaches to the collarbone (clavicle) and sternum, and inserts into the upper arm bone (humerus). It pulls the arm in front of the chest from any position, flexes the shoulder to allow pushing, and lifts the arm forwards. The smaller pectoralis minor lies beneath the pectoralis major and helps lower the shoulder blade.

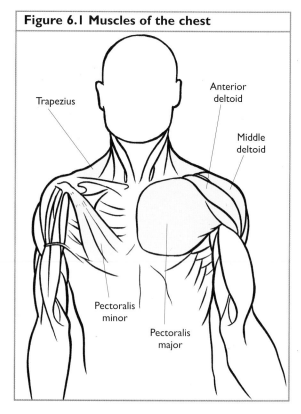

Figure 6.1 Muscles of the chest

Trapezius

Anterior deltoid

Middle deltoid

Pectoralis minor

Pectoralis major

BARBELL BENCH PRESS

Target muscles

Pectoralis major (mid-chest)
Also used: anterior deltoids, triceps

Starting position

1. Lie on your back on a flat bench, ideally with an attached barbell rack. If you have an excessive arch in your back, place your feet on the end of the bench or on a low step.
2. Hold the bar, with your hands just over shoulder-width apart, palms facing forwards.
3. Remove the bar from the barbell rack and position it directly over your chest with your arms fully extended (but not locked).

The movement

1. Slowly lower the bar down to your chest. The bar should touch your upper chest just above your nipple line. Hold for a count of two.

2. Push the bar upwards in a slightly backwards arc so that it ends up over your shoulders.

Tips

- Keep your hips firmly on the bench. If you lift your hips to generate leverage, you will risk lower-back strain.
- Do not bounce the bar off your chest or arch your back – this reduces the amount of chest work and risks injury to the chest muscles.
- Keep your palms facing forwards and your wrists straight.

Variations

WIDE GRIP

Using a grip one and a half times shoulder-width apart places more emphasis on the pectorals (especially the outer part) and less on the triceps.

NARROW GRIP

Using a shoulder-width grip places more emphasis on the triceps and the inner pectorals.

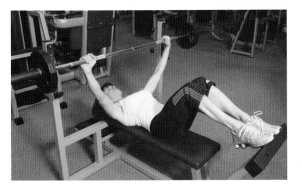

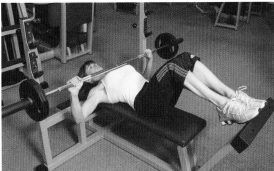

VERTICAL BENCH PRESS MACHINE

Target muscles

Pectoralis major
Also used: anterior deltoids, triceps

Starting position

1. Sit down with your back pressed against the backrest.
2. Adjust the seat height so that the handles are level with your chest. Depress the foot lever to allow you to grab hold of the handles.

The movement

1. Press the handles away from you, fully extending your arms.
2. Hold for a second then return slowly to the starting position.

Tips

- Keep your elbows at the same height throughout the movement.

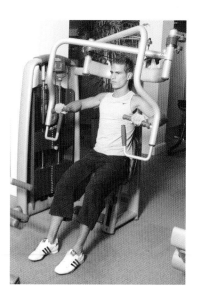
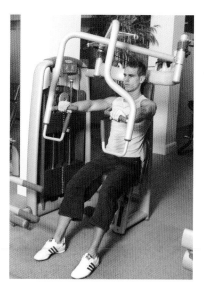

DUMBBELL PRESS

Target muscles

Pectoralis major (mid-chest)
Also used: anterior deltoids, triceps

This exercise develops the chest as well as the barbell bench press, but allows a slightly greater ROM, thus stimulating greater development. It requires more involvement of the stabiliser muscles to balance and control the dumbbells, so you will probably need to use less weight.

Starting position

1. Lie on your back on a flat or incline bench. If you have an excessive arch in your back, place your feet on the end of the bench.

2. Hold a pair of dumbbells, with your palms facing forwards and your arms fully extended, positioned over your shoulders.

The movement

1. Slowly lower the dumbbells down to your armpit area.
2. Hold the position for a count of two, then press the dumbbells back to the starting position.

Tips

• Keep your hips firmly on the bench throughout the movement.
• Lower the dumbbells as far as you can, aiming for a maximum but comfortable stretch.
• Keep the dumbbells over your chest area – do not let them travel back towards your head.

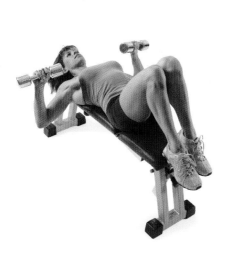

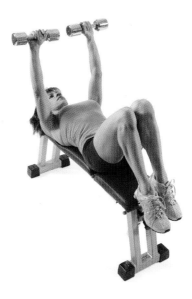

INCLINE BARBELL BENCH PRESS

Target muscles

Pectoralis minor (upper chest)
Also used: anterior deltoids, triceps, pectoralis major

Starting position

1. Lie on an incline bench angled at 30–60 degrees (the steeper the incline, the greater the stress on the upper pectorals and anterior deltoids). Ideally the bench should have an attached barbell rack.
2. Hold the bar with your hands shoulder-width apart, palms facing forwards. Remove the bar from the barbell rack so it is positioned directly over your collarbone with your arms fully extended.

The movement

1. Bend your arms, allowing your elbows to travel out to the sides, and slowly lower the bar down to your chest.
2. The bar should just touch the upper part of your chest beneath your collarbone. Hold for a count of two.
3. Push the bar back to the starting position.

Tips

- Do not arch your back or bounce the bar off your chest as you push the bar upwards. This risks lower-back strain.
- The higher you place the bar on your chest, the greater the work placed on the anterior deltoids rather than the upper chest.

Variation

DECLINE

Set the decline bench about 30 degrees below parallel. The movement is the same, but places more emphasis on your lower chest and triceps.

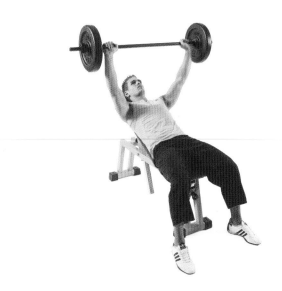
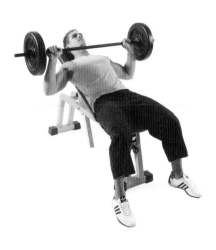

INCLINE DUMBBELL BENCH PRESS

Target muscles

Pectoralis minor (upper chest)
Also used: anterior deltoids, triceps, pectoralis major

Starting position

1. Sit on an incline bench, angled at 30–60 degrees (the steeper the incline, the greater the stress on the upper pectorals and anterior deltoids).
2. Pick up a dumbbell in each hand and place them on your thighs.
3. Lie on the bench, at the same time bringing the dumbbells to shoulder level. Your palms should face forwards.

The movement

1. Press the dumbbells directly over your upper chest until your arms are fully extended. Hold for a count of two.
2. Lower the weights slowly until they are by your shoulders. You should achieve a maximal but comfortable stretch.
3. Pause for a second before pressing them up again.

Tips

- Press the dumbbells in a straight line, not back over your head.
- Do not set the angle of the bench too high otherwise the anterior deltoids will be targeted and take much of the emphasis away from the chest.

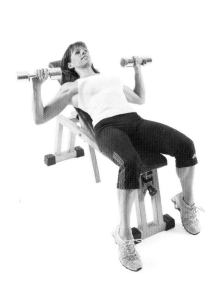

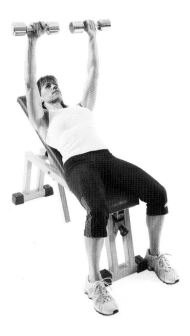

DUMBBELL FLYE

Target muscles

Pectoralis major (mid-chest)
Also used: anterior deltoids, pectoralis minor

Starting position

1. Lie on your back on a flat or incline bench set at 30 degrees with your feet flat on the floor. If you have an excessive arch in your back, place your feet on a step so that your knees are bent at 90 degrees.
2. Hold a dumbbell in each hand and hold them above your chest with your arms extended and palms facing each other. Bend your arms very slightly.

The movement

1. Lower the dumbbell slowly out to your sides in a semi-circular arc. Keep your elbows locked in the slightly bent position throughout the movement.
2. When your upper arms reach shoulder level and you feel a strong stretch in your shoulders, return the dumbbells to the starting position, following the same arc. Do not pause at the bottom of the movement.

Tips

- Maintain the slight bend in your elbows. Don't allow them to bend to 90 degrees as this would turn the movement into a dumbbell press.
- Do not allow your upper arms to go much below shoulder level as this could place excessive stress on the shoulder joints and risk muscle or tendon tears.

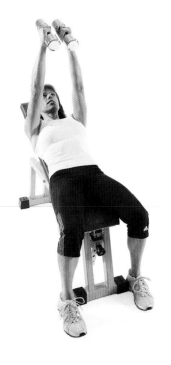

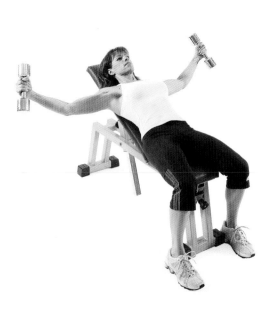

PEC-DECK FLYE

Target muscles

Pectoralis major (mid-chest)
Also used: anterior deltoids, pectoralis minor

Starting position

1. Sit on the seat of the pec-deck machine, ensuring your lower back is pressed against the back support, and adjusting the seat height so that your elbows and shoulders are level with the bottom of the pads.
2. Place your forearms against the pads. Check that your shoulders and elbows form a horizontal line.

The movement

1. Move the pads towards each other until they just touch in front of your chest.
2. Hold for a count of two, then slowly return the pads to the starting position.

Tips

- Contract your pectorals hard at the mid-point.
- Do not curl your shoulders forwards as you bring the pads together.
- Move the pads in a smooth arc – do not jerk them together as this reduces the work on the pectorals.

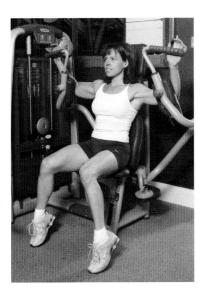
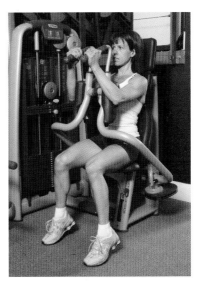

CABLE CROSS-OVER

Target muscles

Pectoralis major (lower and mid-chest)
Also used: anterior deltoids

Starting position

1. Attach the handles to two overhead pulley machines.
2. Hold the handles, palms facing down, and stand midway between the machines with your feet hip-width apart or with one foot in front of the other for balance. Your arms should be fully extended so you achieve a good stretch in your pectorals.
3. Bend forwards slightly from the hips and maintain this position throughout the exercise.

The movement

1. Draw the handles towards each other in an arcing motion, aiming for a point approximately 30 cm in front of your hips.
2. When the handles meet, squeeze your pectorals hard and hold for a count of two.
3. Return the handles slowly to the starting position.

Tips

- Keep your back erect and elbows slightly bent (at 10–15 degrees) throughout the movement.
- Focus on using your chest muscles to perform the movement – do not curl your shoulders forwards as you bring the handles together.
- You can vary the angle at which you pull the handles down to place emphasis on slightly different areas of the chest.

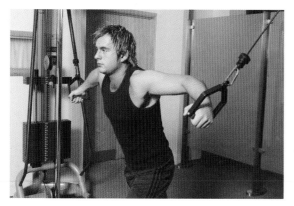
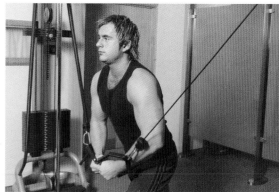

LOW-PULLEY CABLE CROSS-OVER

Target muscles

Pectoralis major (upper and mid-chest), pectoralis minor

Also used: anterior deltoids

Starting position

1. Stand midway between two low-cable machines.
2. Hold the handles with a palms-up grip and stand with your feet hip-width apart or with one foot in front of the other for balance. Your arms should be fully extended so you achieve a good stretch in your pectorals.
3. Bend forwards from the hips about 10–20 degrees.

The movement

1. Pull your arms in and slightly upwards, bringing your hands up under your chest while keeping your elbows in their slightly bent position.
2. Aim for your hands to meet in front of your abs. Hold for a moment.
3. Slowly return the handles to the starting position.

Tips

- Keep your body stationary at all times; the angle in your shoulder should remain the same.
- Keep your arms fairly straight, with your elbows slightly bent throughout the movement.

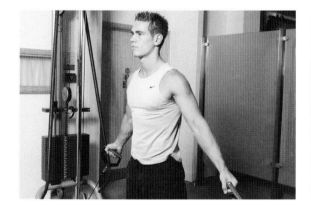
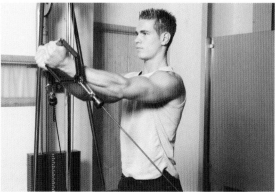

EXERCISE BALL PRESS-UP/ PUSH-UP

Target muscles

Pectoralis major (upper and mid-chest), pectoralis minor, triceps, trunk stabilisers (transverse abdominis and the lumbar multifidus)

Starting position

1. Get in a push-up position, placing the lower part of your shins on top of an exercise ball. Your head, back, hips and knees should be in a straight line.
2. Position your hands just wider than your shoulders, fingers pointing forwards.

The movement

1. Keeping your elbows close to your body, bend your arms until your nose almost touches the floor. Aim your chest between your hands.
2. Straighten your arms back to the starting position. Repeat for reps.

Tips

- Keep your spine in neutral alignment – your head, back, hips and ankles should be in a straight line – and don't let your bottom lift higher than your shoulders.
- Keep your abdominals pulled in – avoid 'swayback'.
- Keep your head in line with your spine – don't allow it to drop.

Variation

To make the movement easier, position the ball just above the knees and keep the movement small. As you get stronger, walk out with your hands until the ball is below the knees and eventually on the lower part of your shins.

To further intensify the move, try lifting one leg a few centimetres from the ball, keeping both legs straight.

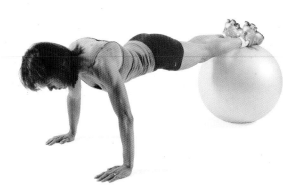
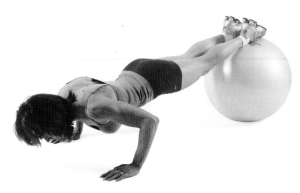

THE SHOULDERS

Shoulder training can change the proportions of your physique. Well-developed shoulders draw more attention to your upper body and create an aesthetically pleasing taper, making your waist appear smaller.

Strong shoulders are advantageous in most sports involving upper body motions. The shoulder muscles are involved in:

- overhead pushing actions – e.g. tumbling and vaulting in gymnastics, and the clean and jerk in weightlifting
- overhead hitting actions – e.g. the tennis serve, the overhead smash in badminton, and overhead hits and blocks in volleyball and basketball
- raising the arms forwards or sideways away from the body – e.g. tennis or squash strokes, and front crawl in swimming.

You need to use a variety of exercises to train your shoulders as there is no single exercise that works the whole area. The shoulders are comprised of three heads (see Figure 7.1), each of which needs to be targeted if you want full and well-balanced development.

If you are prone to shoulder injuries, however, pay attention to your training technique as poor technique can exacerbate any underlying problems.

EXERCISES FOR THE SHOULDERS

Dumbbell press
Overhead press machine
Dumbbell lateral raise
Upright row
Bent-over lateral raise

MUSCLE KNOW-HOW

The shoulder muscle comprises three distinct portions, or heads, collectively known as the deltoids, which is a term derived from the Greek 'delta', owing to their geometrically triangular shape. The deltoids cover the front, side and back of the shoulder, from the scapula (collarbone) to the middle of the upper arm (humerus). Each head serves a particular function. The anterior (front) deltoid lifts the arm forwards and upwards; the medial (outer) deltoid lifts the arm away from the mid-line of the body to the side (abduction); and the posterior (rear) deltoid lifts the arm to the rear or draws the elbow backwards behind the shoulders. Because of their location and function, several of the following exercises that target the deltoids also use muscles in the back and chest (see pp. 62–63 and p. 76).

Figure 7.1 Muscles of the shoulders

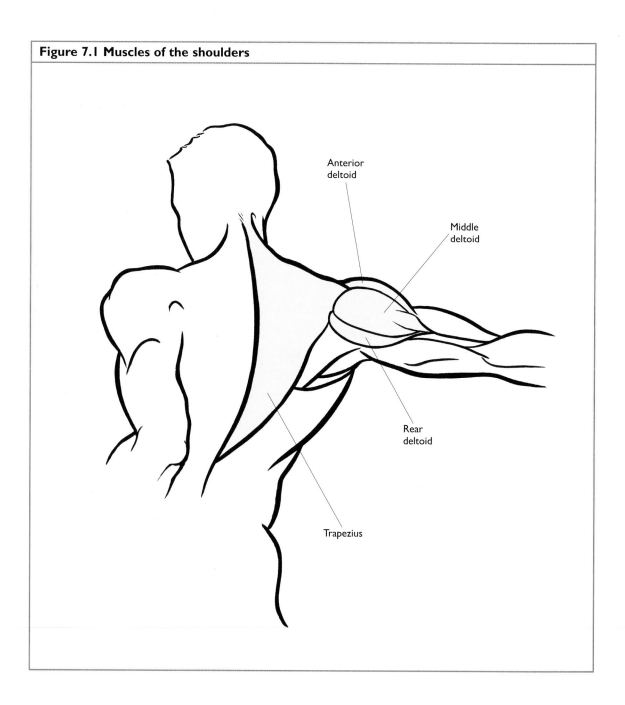

Anterior deltoid

Middle deltoid

Rear deltoid

Trapezius

DUMBBELL SHOULDER PRESS

Target muscles

Anterior and medial deltoids, upper pectoralis major

Also used: triceps, shoulder girdle muscles (trapezius, supraspinatus)

Starting position

1. Sit on the edge of a bench or on an exercise ball, angled at 75–90 degrees so that your lower back is firmly in contact with the bench. If you are using a very heavy weight, use an adjustable bench with an upright back support.
2. Hold a pair of dumbbells, hands facing forwards, level with your shoulders.

The movement

1. Press the dumbbells upwards and inwards until they almost touch over your head.
2. Straighten your arms but do not lock out your elbows. Hold momentarily.
3. Lower the dumbbells slowly back to the starting position.

Tips

- Keep your torso upright – don't lean backwards or arch your spine as you press the bar upwards as this will strain your lower back.
- Hold your abdominal muscles taut to help stabilise your spine or, if you are using a very heavy weight, wear a weightlifting belt.
- Lower the dumbbells until they touch your shoulders – don't shorten the movement.

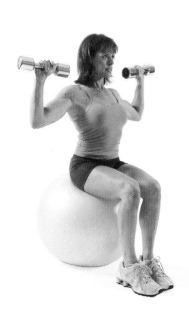
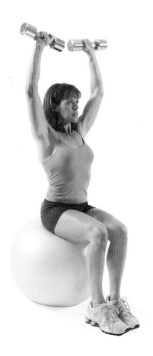

OVERHEAD PRESS MACHINE

Target muscles

Anterior and medial deltoids, upper pectoralis major

Also used: triceps, shoulder girdle muscles (trapezius, supraspinatus)

Starting position

1. Sit in the machine with your feet on the floor and your back against the backrest. Adjust the seat height so that the handles are level with your shoulders.

2. Depress the foot lever to allow you to grasp the handles more comfortably.

The movement

1. Grip the handles and press the weight straight up, extending your arms but not locking out your elbows.
2. Lower the weight slowly and repeat.

Tips

• Keep your back flat against the pad.

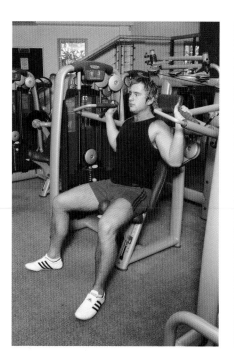

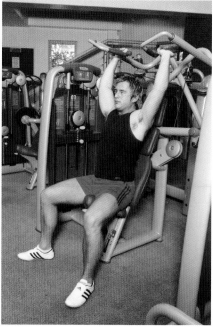

DUMBBELL LATERAL RAISE

Target muscles

Medial deltoids
Also used: trapezius, anterior deltoids

Starting position

1. Stand with your feet hip-width apart. Hold a dumbbell in each hand, arms straight down by your sides, hands facing inwards.

The movement

1. Keeping your elbows very slightly bent (at about 10 degrees), raise the dumbbells out to the sides.
2. Raise them until your elbows and hands are level with your shoulders – i.e. parallel to the floor. Your palms should face the floor. Hold momentarily.
3. Return slowly to the starting position, resisting the weight on the way back down.

Tips

• Your little finger should be higher than your thumb at the top of the movement, as if you were pouring water from a jug.
• Do not swing the dumbbells out or lean back as you raise them. Keep your body very still.
• Lead with your elbows rather than your hands.

Variations

SINGLE ARM LATERAL RAISE

Lateral raises can be performed using one arm at a time. Hold on to an upright support with the other hand to help keep you steady. This allows you to concentrate fully on the movement and helps to prevent you swinging the dumbbells upwards.

CABLE LATERAL RAISE

The movement can be performed using a low pulley machine. You will need to use a lighter weight but this keeps more continuous tension on the deltoids.

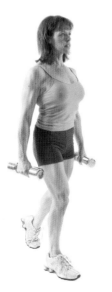

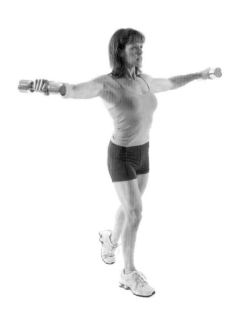

UPRIGHT ROW

Target muscles

Anterior and medial deltoids, trapezius
Also used: biceps, brachioradialis

Starting position

1. Stand with your feet shoulder-width apart.
2. Hold the barbell with your hands about 15 cm apart, palms facing towards your body. The bar should rest against the front of your thighs. The exercise can also be performed on a cable machine, using a short, straight bar attached to the low pulley.

The movement

1. Pull the bar directly upwards towards your chin, bending your elbows out to the sides until the bar is level with your neck.
2. Hold for a count of two, then lower the bar slowly back to the starting position.

Tips

- Keep the bar very close to your body throughout the movement.
- Make sure you do not sway backwards as you lift the bar.
- At the top of the movement your elbows should be level with, or slightly higher than, your hands.
- Lower the bar slowly, resisting the weight.

Variations

WIDE GRIP

Using a shoulder-width grip places more emphasis on the deltoids and less on the trapezius.

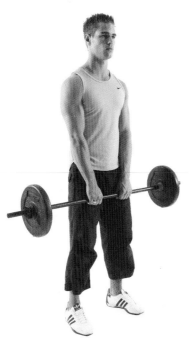
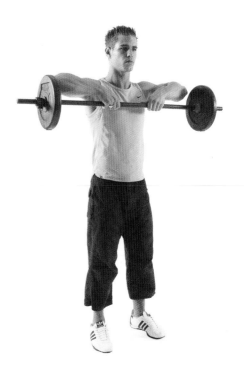

BENT-OVER LATERAL RAISE

Target muscles

Posterior deltoids
Also used: trapezius, upper back muscles

Starting position

1. Sit on the end of a bench with only half of your thighs supported.
2. Place your feet and knees together, bend forwards from the waist and hold a pair of dumbbells underneath your thighs with your palms facing each other.

The movement

1. Draw the dumbbells out to the sides, simultaneously turning your hands so that they face the floor.
2. Raise them until your elbows and hands are level with your shoulders. Hold momentarily.
3. Slowly return to the starting position, resisting the weight on the way down.

Tips

- Your little finger should be higher than your thumb at the top of the movement, as if you are pouring water from a jug.
- Keep your torso still – do not raise your body as you raise the dumbbells.
- Lead with your elbows rather than your hands.
- Keep your elbows bent at about 10 degrees throughout to avoid straining them.

Variation

STANDING BENT-OVER LATERAL RAISE

The movement can be executed from a standing position. Stand with your feet hip-width apart, bend forwards from the hips and hold the dumbbells directly below the shoulders (arms straight).

DUMBBELL LATERAL RAISE ON INCLINE BENCH

The movement can be performed lying face down on an incline bench set at a 30–45-degree angle.

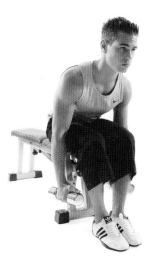

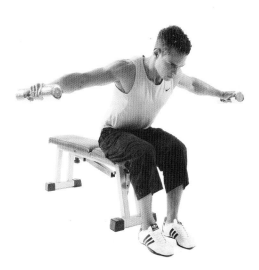

THE ARMS

Arms are the classic showpieces of strength for gym-goers. Like a well-developed chest, they are visible proof of the work you put in at the gym. Even for women, toned, defined arms are enviable assets.

Developing your arm strength will help your performance in many sports. Elbow flexion (bending) and the muscles involved are important when playing forehand strokes in tennis and squash, shooting in hockey, playing a long shot in golf, pulling the body upwards in climbing, grabbing an opponent in rugby and the martial arts, and pushing movements in gymnastics.

The triceps are also involved in numerous upper-body actions, including:

- overhead hitting and throwing movements – e.g. the tennis serve, volleyball spike and basketball shot
- pushing actions – e.g. the shot-put, the chest pass in netball and basketball, throwing a punch in boxing and in the martial arts.

One common mistake is to train only the biceps, thinking this will produce stronger and bigger arms. However, the triceps make up the largest part of the arm muscles (see below) so it is important to devote equal time and effort to triceps training. Many men also use weights that are too heavy in their quest for bigger arms, sacrificing good technique and therefore gaining only minimal results.

EXERCISES FOR THE ARMS

Biceps

Barbell curl
Preacher curl
Dumbbell curl
Incline dumbbell curl
Concentration curl

Triceps

Triceps push-down
Reverse-grip triceps press-down
Bench dip
Lying triceps extension
Triceps kickback
Seated overhead triceps extension

MUSCLE KNOW-HOW

Approximately 60 per cent of the upper-arm muscle mass is comprised of the triceps, 30 per cent is comprised of the biceps brachii, and the remaining 10 per cent comes from the brachialis muscles lying beneath the biceps.

The biceps brachii (see Figure 8.1) originates above the shoulder as two muscles – the short and long heads ('bi' means 'two') – which merge at one insertion point below the elbow. These muscles are involved in flexing your arm (bending your elbow) and rotating (supinating) your forearm. The biceps brachii also assists in other arm and shoulder movements, such as raising the shoulder.

The brachialis runs under the biceps close to your elbow joint. It is also involved in arm flexion and all movements involving a palms-down position (e.g. when performing a reverse curl). The brachioradialis lies on the top side of your forearm, on the same side as your thumb but attaches just past your elbow. It is involved in all arm flexion movements, particularly when you use a neutral, or thumbs-up, grip.

The triceps brachii (see Figure 8.2) makes up the entire back of the arm. It has three distinct heads: the inner (long) head, the medial head and outer (lateral) head. The medial head is located on the back inner side of the arm, fairly close to the elbow. The lateral head, which works progressively harder as the weight increases, is located on the back outer side of the arm. The long inner head, lying between the medial and lateral heads higher up on the arm, gives the familiar horseshoe appearance to the outside upper arm. Whereas the medial and lateral heads only cross the elbow joint, the long head crosses both the shoulder and elbow joints.

The collective function of the triceps brachii is to partially or fully straighten the arm from a bent position. While it is difficult to isolate its individual heads, different exercises place greater emphasis on different areas. For example, the long head is best stimulated when your arm is raised overhead (e.g. in lying triceps extensions).

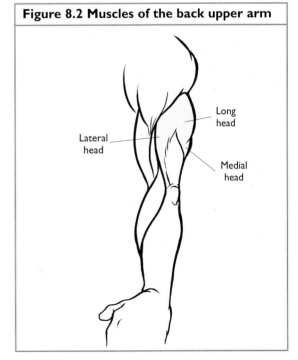

Figure 8.1 Muscles of the front upper arm

Biceps brachii

Brachialis

Pronator teres

Brachioradialis

Figure 8.2 Muscles of the back upper arm

Lateral head

Long head

Medial head

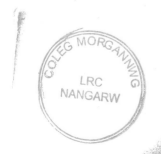

BARBELL CURL

Target muscles

Biceps brachii, brachialis
Also used: brachioradialis

Starting position

1. Stand with your feet hip-width apart.
2. Hold a barbell with your hands shoulder-width apart, palms facing forwards.
3. The bar should rest against your thighs and your arms should be fully extended.

The movement

1. Bend your elbows as you curl the bar up in a smooth arc towards your shoulders. Keep your upper arms fixed by the sides of your body.
2. Hold for a count of two, then slowly lower the bar back to the starting position.

Tips

- Do not move your upper arms or elbows at any point of the movement.
- Keep your body absolutely still – make sure you do not lean back or swing the bar up as this will strain the back and reduce the work on the biceps.
- Keep your wrists locked.
- Lower the bar under control until your arms are fully extended – shortening or rushing the downward phase will reduce the effectiveness of the exercise.

Variations

EZ-BAR CURL

Arm curls can be performed using an EZ-bar instead of a straight bar. This reduces the stress on the wrists, although it puts the biceps in a bio-mechanically weaker position so they receive less stimulation.

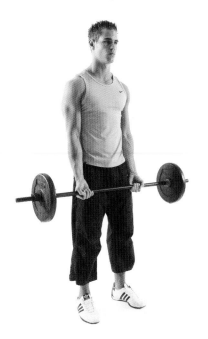
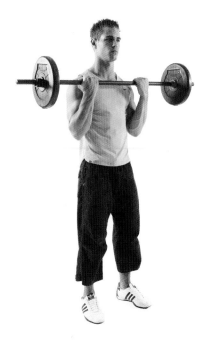

PREACHER CURL

Target muscles

Biceps brachii, brachialis
Also used: brachioradialis

Starting position

1. Adjust the seat on the preacher curl bench to the right height – your armpits should rest over the top edge of the pad. If a preacher bench isn't available, simply use an incline bench and perform the exercise with a dumbbell one arm at a time.
2. Hold a dumbbell or barbell with your hands shoulder-width apart, palms facing forwards.
3. Your arms should be fully extended.

The movement

1. Bend your elbows as you curl the barbell or dumbbell up in a smooth arc towards your shoulders, stopping about 20–30 cm short of your shoulders.
2. Hold for a count of two, then slowly lower the bar back to the starting position.

Tips

- Keep your shoulders back and relaxed – avoid leaning forwards as you curl the bar up or the emphasis will shift from your biceps to your shoulders.
- Keep your body still and your wrists locked.
- Lower the bar until your arms are fully extended – shortening the downward phase will reduce the effectiveness of the exercise.

Variations

EZ-BAR PREACHER CURL

Preacher curls can be performed using an EZ-bar instead of a straight bar. This reduces the stress on the wrists although it puts the biceps in a biomechanically weaker position so they receive less stimulation.

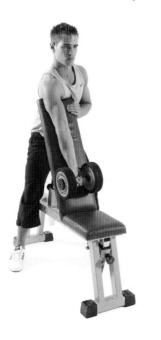
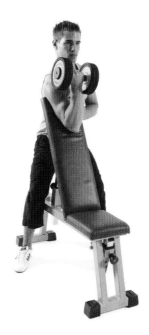

DUMBBELL CURL

Target muscles

Biceps brachii, brachialis
Also used: brachioradialis

Starting position

1. Stand with your feet hip-width apart or sit on the end of a bench or on an exercise ball.
2. Hold a pair of dumbbells, palms facing in towards your body.
3. Your arms should be fully extended.

The movement

1. Curl one dumbbell up at a time in a smooth arc towards your shoulders, rotating your forearm so that your palm faces your shoulder at the top of the movement.

2. Hold for a count of two, then slowly lower the dumbbell back to the starting position.
3. Repeat with the other arm and continue alternating arms.

Tips

- Curl the dumbbells up slowly – do not swing them.
- Keep your upper arms fixed by the sides of your body.
- Keep your body absolutely still – make sure you do not sway backwards.
- Make sure you straighten your arms fully when you lower the dumbbells; do not shorten the downward phase.

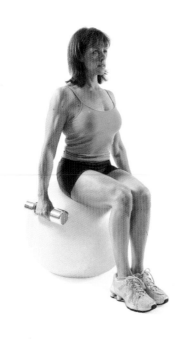 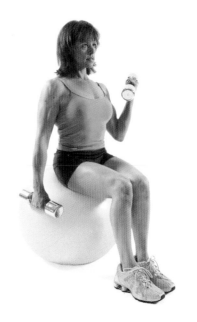

INCLINE DUMBBELL CURL

Target muscles

Biceps brachii, brachialis
Also used: brachioradialis

Starting position

1. Sit on an incline bench with your back and shoulders pressed firmly against it.
2. Hold a pair of dumbbells by your sides, palms facing inwards.
3. Your arms should be fully extended and hang downwards.

The movement

1. Slowly curl one dumbbell towards your shoulder, rotating your forearm so that your palm faces your shoulder at the top of the movement.
2. Hold for a count of two, then slowly lower the dumbbell back to the starting position.
3. Repeat with the other arm and continue alternating arms.

Tips

• The lower the incline, the greater the stretch on the upper biceps.
• Keep your head back against the bench throughout the movement.
• Keep your elbows pointed down and back as best as possible.

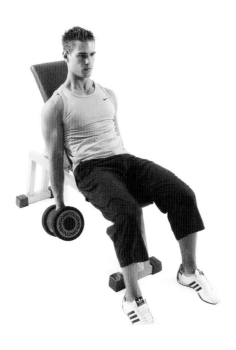
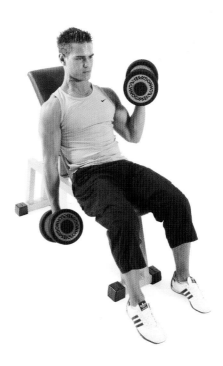

CONCENTRATION CURL

Target muscles

Biceps brachii, brachialis
Also used: brachioradialis

Starting position

1. Sit on a bench with your legs fairly wide apart.
2. Hold a dumbbell with one hand and brace that arm against the inside of the same thigh.
3. Your arm should be fully extended and your palm should be facing the opposite thigh.

The movement

1. Curl the dumbbell up slowly in a smooth arc towards your shoulder.
2. Squeeze your biceps hard at the top of the movement, hold for a count of two and then slowly lower the dumbbell back to the starting position.

Tips

- Make sure you curl the dumbbell to your shoulder and do not move your shoulder to the dumbbell. Keep your shoulder back and relaxed.
- Do not lean backwards.
- Keep your upper arm fixed.
- Make sure you straighten your arms fully when you lower the dumbbells; do not shorten the downward phase.

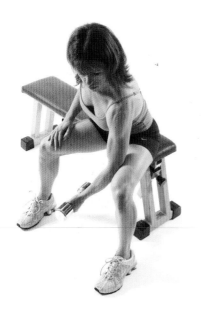
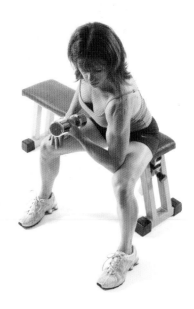

TRICEPS PUSH-DOWN

Target muscles

Triceps (especially the outer and medial heads)
Also used: brachioradialis

Starting position

1. Attach a short, angled or straight bar to the overhead cable of a lat machine. Alternatively, use a short rope attachment.
2. Place your hands on the bar, palms facing downwards.
3. Bring the bar down until your elbows are at your sides and bent at about 90 degrees.

The movement

1. Keeping your upper arms close to your body, press the bar down, moving only your forearms, until your arms are fully extended.
2. Hold for a count of two, then slowly return the bar to the starting position.

Tips

- Keep your elbows fixed firmly at your sides throughout the movement.
- Do not lean too far forwards.
- Keep your wrists locked and your palms facing you.

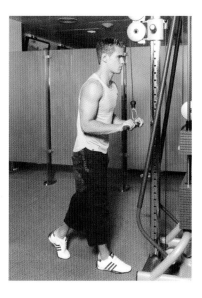
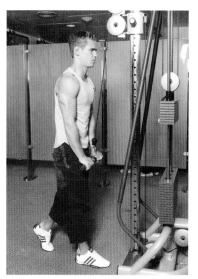

REVERSE-GRIP TRICEPS PRESS-DOWN

Target muscles

Triceps (especially the lateral head)
Also used: brachioradialis

Starting position

1. Stand in front of a high-pulley cable machine. Position one leg slightly in front of the other.
2. Grasp the stirrup handle with a palms-up grip.
3. Bring the bar down until your elbow is bent at an angle of about 90 degrees.

The movement

1. Press the handle down, until your arm is fully extended. Keep your elbow in place at your side.
2. Hold for a count of two, then slowly return the handle to the starting position. Repeat for reps then switch arms.

Tips

• Keep your upper arm and elbow locked in to the side of your body.
• Make sure you fully extend your arm and lock out your elbows at the bottom of the press-down.

Variation

This exercise can be performed with a short, straight bar.

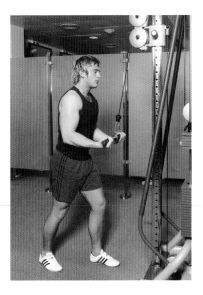
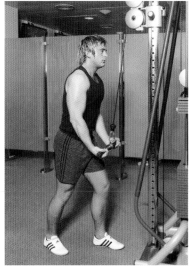

BENCH DIP

Target muscles

Triceps (especially the outer and medial heads)

Starting position

1. Position two benches or steps about the length of your legs apart.
2. Place your hands shoulder-width apart, fingers facing forwards, on the edge of one bench.
3. Place your heels on the other bench so that your legs form a straight bridge between the two benches.

The movement

1. Bend your elbows and lower your body until your elbows form an angle of 90 degrees.
2. Hold for a count of two, then straighten your arms to bring you back to the starting position.

Tips

- Keep your back close to the bench.
- Do not lock or snap out your elbows at the top of the movement.
- Keep your elbows directed backwards during both the lowering and raising phases.
- Do not shorten the downward phase.
- Keep the movement slow – do not rush the reps.

Variations

EASIER

Place your feet flat on the floor instead of on a bench.

ADVANCED

Place a weight disc across your lap to increase the resistance.

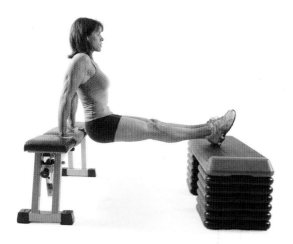
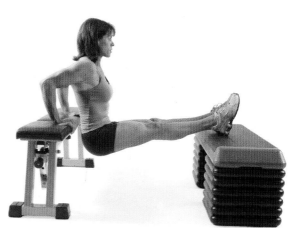

LYING TRICEPS EXTENSION

Target muscles

Triceps (especially the long inner and medial heads)
Also used: brachioradialis

Starting position

1. Lie on your back on a flat bench. If you have an excessive arch in your back, place your feet on the end of the bench or on a low step.
2. Hold a barbell or EZ-bar with your hands slightly less than shoulder-width apart, palms facing forwards.
3. The bar should be positioned directly over your head with your arms fully extended.

The movement

1. Keeping your upper arms absolutely stationary, bend your elbows as you lower the bar until it just touches your forehead.

2. Hold for a count of two, then straighten your arms back to the starting position.

Tips

- For maximum muscle development, straighten your arms fully at the end of the movement.
- Keep your elbows perfectly still – do not allow them to move out to the sides, or backwards with the bar.
- Keep your lower back firmly pressed down on the bench.
- Lower the bar as far back as you safely can to achieve the greatest ROM.

Variations

LYING DUMBBELL TRICEPS EXTENSION

Use a dumbbell instead of a barbell and place your hands against the inner side of one of the end plates. You may also perform this exercise holding a pair of dumbbells, palms facing each other or a single dumbbell, one arm at a time.

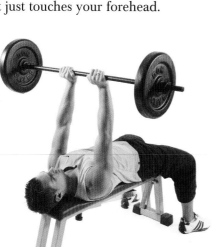

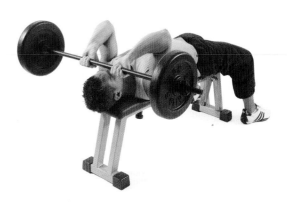

TRICEPS KICKBACK

> ### Target muscles
>
> Triceps (especially the outer and medial heads)

Starting position

1. Hold a dumbbell in one hand.
2. Bend forwards from the waist until your torso is parallel to the floor.
3. Place your other hand and knee on a bench to stabilise yourself – your back should be flat and horizontal.
4. Bend the working arm to 90 degrees at the elbow and bring it up so that your upper arm is parallel to and close to the side of your body, and the dumbbell is hanging straight down below the elbow.

The movement

1. Keeping your elbow stationary, extend your arm backwards until your arm is straight and horizontal.
2. Hold for a count of two, then slowly return to the starting position.

Tips

- Extend your arm under control – do not swing the dumbbell back.
- Keep your upper arm fixed – only your forearm moves.
- Keep your lower back flat and still.
- Use a relatively light weight as the exercise is harder to perform than many people imagine.

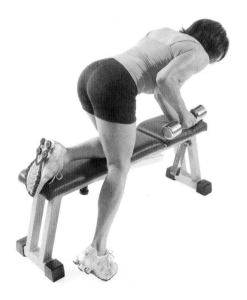

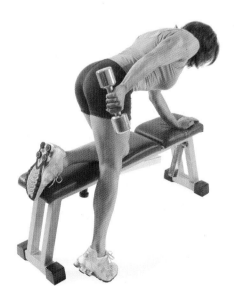

SEATED OVERHEAD TRICEPS EXTENSION

Target muscles
Triceps

Starting position

1. Sit on a bench, feet flat on the floor.
2. Grasp one end of a dumbbell with both hands, palms up, and raise it above your head, arms extended.

The movement

1. Keeping your upper arms stationary, slowly lower the dumbbell behind your head until you feel a stretch in your triceps.
2. Hold for a moment, then press the weight back up until your arms are fully extended.

Tips

- Keep your upper arms vertical so your elbows point directly overhead at all times. This will ensure the focus is kept on the triceps and does not involve the shoulders.
- Lock your elbows in the top overhead position (but make sure your arms are in a vertical line). This produces a stronger contraction of the triceps.
- Keep your torso erect throughout the movement – make sure you use a weight that isn't too heavy.

Variation

ONE-ARM OVERHEAD EXTENSION

This exercise can be done one arm at a time, holding a dumbbell in one hand.

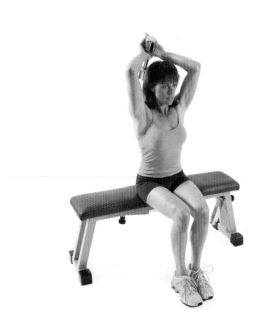
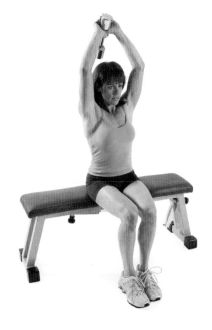

THE ABDOMINALS

Well-defined abdominals are the product of hard training, careful eating and low body-fat levels. If you are after a rippling six-pack, you need to reduce your abdominal fat layer for the muscles to show through. Increasing their size alone through exercise will not be enough. For these muscles to become visible, men need to have 10–12 per cent body fat and women need to have 15–18 per cent body fat – ranges that are below those considered healthy among the general population (see p. 201) but that are compatible with improved sports performance.

Strong abdominals help you perform virtually every strength training exercise and sports movement, and improve core stability. Abdominal training is also important for the prevention of lower-back injuries, since these muscles help stabilise the pelvis which, in turn, helps maintain proper spine alignment. You should add a lower-back exercise such as back extensions to your abdominal routine to help balance abdominal strength.

EXERCISES FOR THE ABDOMINALS

Crunch
Exercise ball crunch
Reverse crunch
Oblique crunch
Alternate twisting exercise ball crunch
Hip thrust
Side crunch
Hanging leg raise
Exercise ball pull-in
Plank
Side bridge
Exercise ball jack-knife

MUSCLE KNOW-HOW

The abdominals are comprised of four main muscle groups:
1. the rectus abdominis (the 'six-pack' muscle), running from your pubic bone to your lower ribs, which flexes the torso so the rib cage moves towards the pelvis
2. the external obliques, running diagonally from the lower ribs to the opposite hip, which bend the torso sideways and rotate it to the opposite side when flexing forwards
3. the internal obliques, running in the opposite direction to the external obliques, which help the rectus abdominis bend the torso forwards,

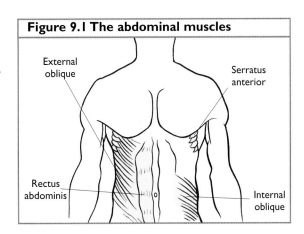

Figure 9.1 The abdominal muscles

External oblique

Serratus anterior

Rectus abdominis

Internal oblique

as well as rotating it to the same side to which they are located

4. the transverse abdominis, a deep, flat sheath of muscle running across the torso, which acts as a muscular girdle to support the contents of the abdomen.

Back strain?

Weak abdominals are often associated with back problems. This is because slack abdominal muscles can become overstretched and this, when combined with tight hip flexors (connecting the thigh bone to the lower vertebrae), can cause the pelvis to tilt forwards (lordosis) creating an excessive arch in the lower back and potential back pain. Strong abdominals support and stabilise the pelvis and lower back. Strengthening these muscles (and stretching the hip flexors) will eliminate excessive arching in the lower back, give good posture and minimise potential back problems.

Maintain a neutral alignment of the spine at all times – during everyday activities as well as when exercising – by keeping the natural 'S' contour of the spine. Your ears, shoulders, hips, knees and ankles should form a perfectly straight line when viewed from the side. This neutral position distributes the load more evenly and minimises stress to the vertebrae and discs of the spine.

Technique tips

Gadgets and machines are unnecessary – you can develop great abdominals from the basic exercises that require nothing more than the floor and perhaps an exercise ball.

The secret to effective abdominal exercising is mental focus and technique. You should concentrate on each part of the movement, keeping it slow and controlled. Don't worry about how far you are moving – it's the feel that is most important. The most common error is to perform the movements too fast, aiming for a high number of repetitions. High repetitions will not work the important FT muscle fibres that give your abdominals good shape, nor will they increase definition or melt away fat.

Although your spine flexes during many of the exercises, keep your neck, head and shoulders in alignment; don't press your chin into your chest – imagine you are holding an apple under your chin and keep a gap of that size there at all times when performing the exercises.

The abdominals are the same as any other muscle and should be trained in the same fashion: no more than every other day and no more than 12–15 repetitions per set. So slow down, visualise your abdominals working and focus on feeling the contraction through the full ROM. When it starts to hurt (not to be confused with actual pain), take a short rest, then complete the exercise or move on to the next.

The sit-up controversy

The traditional feet-restrained sit-up is not recommended as it can put stress on the lower back and aggravate back pain. This is because the psoas – a hip flexor, which attaches to the fourth and fifth lumbar vertebrae – is involved in the movement (even if your knees are bent). When you bring your chest towards your hips from a lying position the hip flexors initially do most of the work. Only in the last part of the movement do the abdominals contract. So, not only is the movement largely ineffective for the abs, it can also put stress on the lower back. Keep your knees slightly bent and feet unsecured to minimise hip flexor involvement when doing abdominal exercises.

CRUNCH

Starting position

1. Lie flat on your back, either on the floor or on an abdominal bench, with your knees bent over your hips and your ankles touching. If you are on the floor, rest your feet on a bench with your knees bent at 90 degrees.
2. Place your hands lightly by the sides of your head or across your chest.
3. Press your lower back to the floor or bench.

The movement

1. Use your abdominal strength to raise your head and shoulders from the floor or bench. You should only come up about 10 cm and your lower back should remain on the floor or bench.
2. Hold this contracted position for a count of two.

3. Let your body uncurl slowly back to the starting position.

Tips

- Focus on moving your ribs towards your hips.
- Do not pull your head with your hands – keep your elbows out and relaxed.
- Exhale as you contract your abdominals.

Variation

EASIER

To make the movement easier, place your feet flat on the floor, knees bent at about 60 degrees, or cross your arms over your chest.

HARDER

To make the exercise harder, stretch your arms overhead, crossing your palms.

STRAIGHT-LEG CRUNCH

Perform the movement with your legs straight up in the air. This requires your lower abs to work isometrically with your arms in front of you, while you curl up, reaching towards your toes.

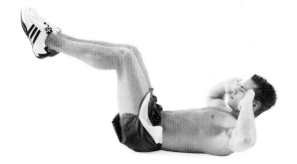
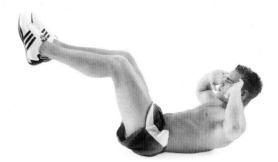

EXERCISE BALL CRUNCH

Target muscles

Rectus abdominis (mainly upper portion), transverse abdominis

Starting position

1. Sit on top of an exercise ball, feet on the floor. Slide forwards, rolling the ball under your bottom until your lower back is centred on top of the ball.
2. Cross your arms over your chest or, to make the exercise harder, place your hands by the sides of your head.

The movement

1. Making sure that you move only your upper body and that your lower back remains in contact with the ball, slowly raise your torso.

2. Hold the position for a count of two, then lower yourself back to the starting position.

Tips

- When you lower yourself back down, keep the movement controlled.
- Do not let your upper body arch backwards or your head flop back over the ball.
- To make the movement harder, bring your whole body higher up on to the top of the ball.

Variation

To make the exercise harder, extend your arms behind your head. Or hold a dumbbell in front of your chest or behind your head. Make sure you start with a light weight.

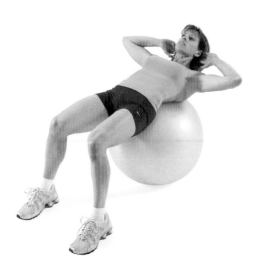
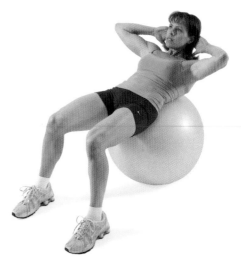

REVERSE CRUNCH

Target muscles

Rectus abdominis (mainly lower part)

Starting position

1. Lie flat on your back on the floor or on a bench with your knees bent over your hips and your ankles touching (as for crunches).
2. Place your arms on the floor alongside your body, palms flat on the floor, or hold on to the sides of the bench.
3. Press your lower back to the floor or bench.

The movement

1. Curl your hips slowly off the floor, aiming your knees towards your chest. Your hips should raise no more than 10 cm.
2. Hold for a count of two.
3. Slowly lower your hips to the starting position, maintaining constant tension in your abdominals.

Tips

• This should be a controlled, deliberate movement. Do not jerk, swing or bounce your hips off the floor; curl up one vertebra at a time.
• Do not allow your abdominals to relax at the top of the movement or while you are uncurling.
• Exhale as you contract your abdominals.

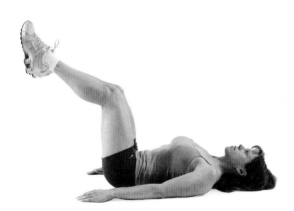
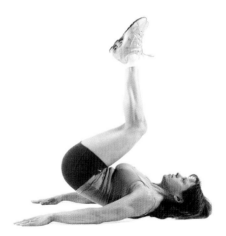

OBLIQUE CRUNCH

Starting position

1. Lie on your back with your knees bent and feet either resting on a bench or flat on the floor.
2. Place your hands by the side of your head.

The movement

1. Lift your right shoulder diagonally, aiming it towards your left knee.
2. Hold for two counts, then slowly return to your starting position.
3. After completing the required number of repetitions, repeat the exercise on the other side.

Tips

- Imagine your rib cage rotating to the side as you curl up.
- Lead with your shoulder rather than your elbow.
- Make sure you lower your upper body slowly back to the floor.
- Do not twist your head, only your torso.
- Exhale as you contract your abdominals.

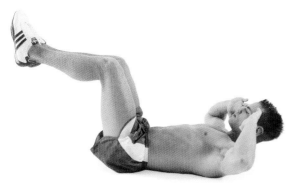
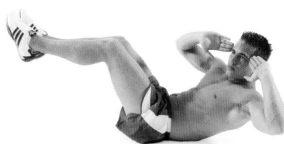

ALTERNATE TWISTING EXERCISE BALL CRUNCH

Target muscles

Internal and external obliques, rectus abdominis

Starting position

1. Sit on top of an exercise ball, feet on the floor. Slide forwards, rolling the ball under your bottom until your lower back is centred on top of the ball.
2. Place your hands by the sides of your head.

The movement

1. Slowly raise your upper body, rotating one elbow towards the opposite knee.
2. Pause briefly as you contract your obliques then return to the starting position, rotating your body back to its original position.
3. Repeat to the opposite side.

Tips

- Lead with your shoulder rather than your elbow.
- Don't pull on your head – use your abs and obliques to raise and rotate your torso.

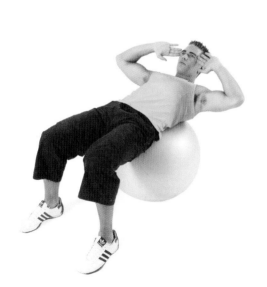
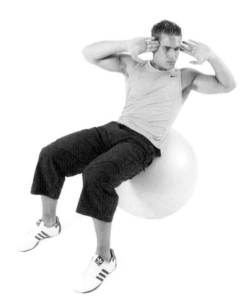

HIP THRUST

Target muscles

Rectus abdominis (mainly lower part)

Starting position

1. Lie flat on your back with your arms on the floor alongside your body, palms down.
2. Lift your legs perpendicular to the floor. They should be straight.

The movement

1. Use your abs to lift your hips only a few centimetres off the floor, aiming your heels towards the ceiling.

2. Hold for a count of two.
3. Slowly lower your hips to the starting position, maintaining constant tension in your abdominals.

Tips

- The range of motion is very limited – your hips should raise no more than 10 cm.
- Keep the movement slow and controlled – do not jerk, swing or bounce your hips off the floor.
- To make it easier, bend your knees at about 60 degrees.

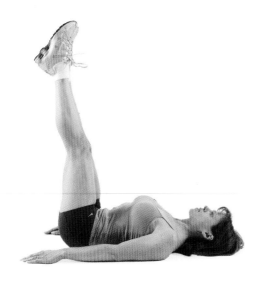
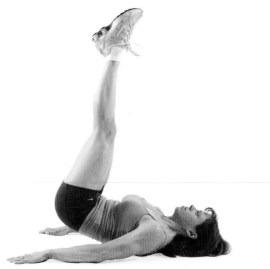

SIDE CRUNCH

Target muscles

Internal and external obliques, rectus abdominis

Starting position

1. Lie on the floor or on an abdominal bench, on your side with your knees slightly bent.
2. Place your top arm behind your head.

The movement

1. Exhale slowly as you raise your head and shoulders a short distance off the floor or bench, aiming your ribs towards your top hip.

2. Hold for a count of two, then breathe in as you return to the starting position.
3. Repeat for the required number of repetitions, then perform the exercise on your other side.

Tips

- Aim to reduce the space between your ribs and hips.
- Do not worry if you don't reach up very far – concentrate on feeling the movement.
- Keep your head in line with your body – don't jerk it upwards.

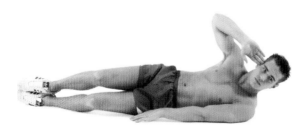

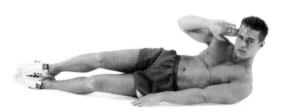

HANGING LEG RAISE

Target muscles

Rectus abdominis (especially lower portion), hip flexors

Starting position

1. Hang from a high bar with your hands shoulder-width apart. (You may use wrist or elbow straps for support.)
2. Your arms should be fully extended and your lower back slightly arched.

The movement

1. Take your legs slightly behind your body.
2. Keeping your legs almost straight, exhale and raise them upwards as high as possible. Ideally they should come just above the level of your hips. Focus on curling your hips towards your rib cage.
3. Hold for a count of two, then slowly return your legs to the starting position.

Tips

- Do not swing your knees up or use the momentum of your legs – use the strength of your abdominals to move your hips and legs.
- For maximal results, raise your legs to approximately 30–45 degrees to the horizontal. The abs shorten only when your legs go past parallel – below this point, they hold a static contraction as the hip flexors raise the legs.
- To make the exercise easier, bend your knees to reduce the resistance.

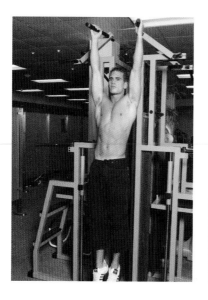
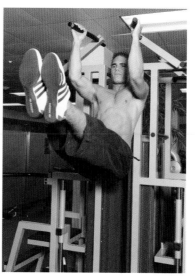

EXERCISE BALL PULL-IN

Target muscles

Rectus abdominis, transverse abdominis

Starting position

1. Get in a push-up position, placing the lower part of your shins on top of an exercise ball.
2. Your head, back, hips and knees should be in a straight line.

The movement

1. Slowly pull your knees in towards your chest, allowing the ball to roll forwards under your ankles.

2. Hold for a moment with your abs contracted. Return to the starting position by straightening your legs and rolling the ball away from your body.

Tips

Try tucking your chin into your chest during the movement.

Variation

TWISTING EXERCISE BALL PULL-IN

Target your obliques by pulling your right knee towards your left side instead of pulling your knees in straight. Straighten, then repeat to the opposite side.

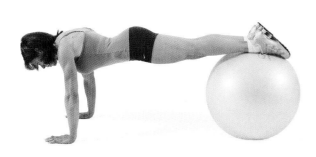

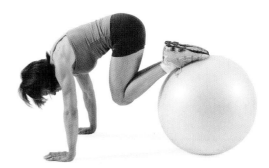

PLANK

Target muscles

Rectus abdominis, transverse abdominis

Starting position

1. Lie face down on the floor with your hips and legs in contact with the floor, your upper body raised and supported on your forearms.
2. Your elbows should be directly under your shoulders by the sides of your body, palms down.

The movement

1. Lift your hips so that only your forearms and toes are on the floor. Keep your spine in neutral alignment – your head, back, hips and ankles should be in a straight line.

2. Hold for 60–120 seconds, then slowly lower back to the starting position.

Tips

- Keep your abs held in during the hold to protect your back.
- Check your neck, torso and legs are in a straight line.
- Make sure you don't let your bottom lift higher than your shoulders.
- Keep your shoulders pulled down and try to lengthen the distance between your shoulders and ears.

Variation

For a more advanced version, perform the plank in a push-up position, supporting your body weight on your hands instead of your forearms. Make it more challenging by raising one leg without letting the hips move. Hold, lower and repeat with the other leg.

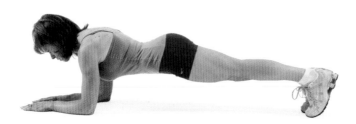

SIDE BRIDGE

Target muscles

Obliques, transverse abdominis

Starting position

1. Lie on your right side, propping your body up on your elbow. Your elbow should be under your shoulder.
2. Your legs should be straight.

The movement

1. Lift your hips so that only your right forearm and right ankle are in contact with the floor.
2. Your body should be a straight line. Keep your spine long and in neutral alignment.

3. Hold for 5–10 seconds, then slowly lower back to the starting position. Repeat for reps, then switch sides.

Tips

- Lift your hips as high as possible without rolling forwards or back.
- Keep your hips stacked on top of each other.
- Keep your neck neutral and in line with your spine.

Variation

To make the exercise harder, support your upper body on your hand instead of your forearm. You can raise your left (top) arm to the ceiling.

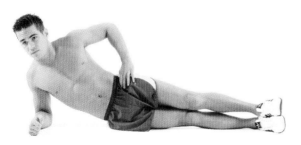
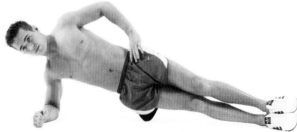

EXERCISE BALL JACK-KNIFE

Target muscles

Rectus abdominis, transverse abdominis

Starting position

1. Get in a push-up position, resting the lower part of your shins on top of an exercise ball.
2. Make sure your arms are straight, and that your back and legs are straight.

The movement

1. Pull your lower body slowly in towards your hands, allowing the ball to roll forwards and raising your hips as high as you can.
2. Pause, contracting your abs hard, then roll the ball back to the starting position.

Tips

• This exercise requires considerable core strength and upper body strength, so practise the movement with a spotter first.
• Keep the movement smooth and controlled.
• Roll the ball in as close to your hands as possible, tuck your chin in – your torso should be almost vertical.

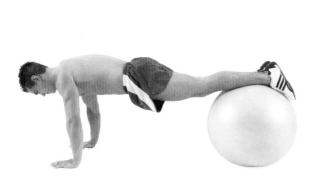
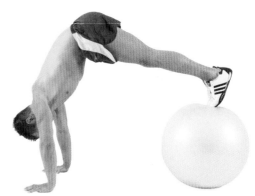

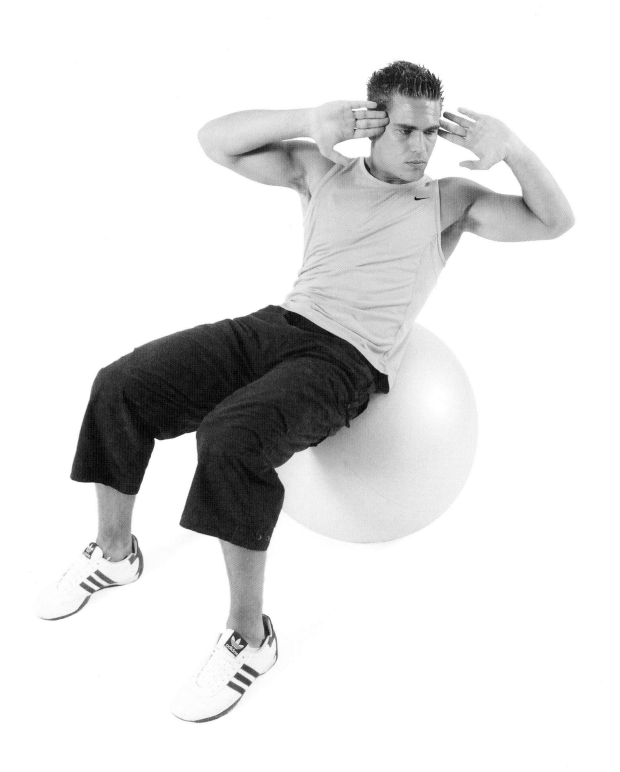

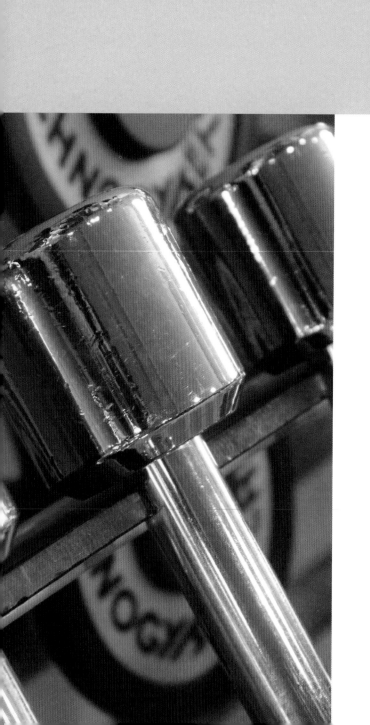

PART **THREE**

PLANNING A PROGRAMME

Now you're ready to plan your programme. Like any great journey, you need to have clear goals and be well equipped to deal with the rigours that lie ahead. In the following chapters, you'll learn how to find a good gym, how to set goals and motivate yourself and how to design the most effective training programme for you – just about everything you need to embark on your trip!

GETTING STARTED

10

There are several important decisions you need to make before embarking on a weights programme, not least where you are going to train, what equipment you will use and what workout gear you will need. This chapter covers these key areas and helps you make the right decisions for you.

HOME OR GYM TRAINING?

The decision whether to join a gym or train at home will depend on your fitness goals and the constraints of your lifestyle. Ask yourself the following questions.
- What are your fitness goals?
- How much time can you spend training?
- How much money do you want to spend?
- How good are you at motivating yourself?
- How sociable are you?
- How good are you at achieving your goals?
- How far are you prepared to travel to a gym?
Table 10.1 summarises the advantages and disadvantages of training at home or in a gym.

Designing your home gym

Create a designated area in your home to train – a basement workout room, the garage – somewhere that provides a good atmosphere to train in, similar to a gym.
- Buy good-quality equipment – try it out before you buy.
- Keep it as a home gym – don't use it for storage.
- Create a gym atmosphere – play music, hang mirrors and pictures on the wall and put rubber mats on the floor to prevent damage from the weights.
- Make your home gym a 'real' gym.

Checklist for finding a good gym

If, however, you decide you would like to join a gym, you will need to consider the following points.

TRAVELLING DISTANCE AND TIME

Decide how far you are prepared to travel. If the journey takes you more than 15–20 minutes you are unlikely to visit the gym regularly in the long term once the initial novelty has worn off.

TYPE OF EQUIPMENT

Is there a good range of equipment to suit your needs? If you want to build mass, you will need plenty of free weights (see below), benches and racks. If you are more interested in general fitness and toning, you may prefer a greater range of machines and lighter free weights.

STANDARD AND SAFETY OF EQUIPMENT

Good equipment does not need to be state-of-the-art shiny machinery. Check that the equipment is well maintained with no broken or loose attachments, and that it is cleaned and tested regularly.

GYM LAYOUT

The gym should be well ventilated and well laid out, with enough space between equipment to prevent accidents and overcrowding.

Table 10.1	The pros and cons of training at home and at the gym		
GYM		**HOME**	
Advantages	*Disadvantages*	*Advantages*	*Disadvantages*
• Greater variety of equipment, including free weights, machines and cardiovascular equipment • Instructors on hand to ensure that you are training correctly, offering advice and helping you develop your training programme • More motivating to train with other people and in a sociable club atmosphere • Spotter or training partners allow you to train harder and reduce the risk of injury or accidents • You may have access to other fitness facilities that would complement your strength training, such as a swimming pool and fitness classes	• Membership fees can be expensive, although once you've paid you may be more motivated to stick to your programme and less likely to skip workouts • Overcrowding, particularly during peak times, may be a problem • More time-consuming to travel to a gym	• You are training in the privacy of your own home • You can train when you like • You don't have to travel to the gym, so it can save time	• Initial outlay for home gym equipment can be expensive • Your budget and available space will probably limit you to only the basics • Your initial enthusiasm may wear off fast and, unless you set aside specific times to work out, you can always find other things to do instead • Unless you train with a partner or personal trainer, it can be difficult to motivate yourself and push yourself hard enough in a home environment to achieve significant gains • Greater risk of accident or injury unless training with a partner or personal trainer

ATMOSPHERE AND MOTIVATION

The gym environment should be motivating for you as an individual. Some gyms are very busy and noisy, others are quieter; it is important to train in an atmosphere that suits your temperament. Try to get an idea of the type of members who train there – are they serious bodybuilders or general fitness trainers, sociable or quiet?

INSTRUCTION

Check that the instructors are professionally qualified. Most instructors in the UK will have a certificate (minimum NVQ Level 2) in fitness training or weight training, or hold a degree in sports science or a related subject.

ARRANGE A TRIAL WORKOUT

Most gyms will be happy to arrange a trial workout. Arrange to visit at the same time as you plan to exercise so you can see whether the gym becomes overcrowded and you will need to queue for equipment.

COST

Make sure you find out the true cost of joining a gym. Some require an initial non-refundable joining fee, plus an annual or monthly membership subscription. Others may allow you to pay for each workout – multiply this by the number of times you intend to train per year. Also make sure you are clear about what the membership buys you, whether you need to pay extra for other facilities, and ask about different payment methods. Find out whether any discounts are available (e.g. off-peak membership).

FREE WEIGHTS OR MACHINES?

Free weights and machines offer different benefits and can both be included in a strength training programme.

The case for free weights

When you perform an exercise with free weights, you not only use the specific muscles involved in the lift (the prime movers) but the rest of the body gets involved too. You have to work to balance and control the weight using another set of muscles that acts to stabilise your body and keep the bar or dumbbells in the correct trajectory. This helps develop greater coordination skills and facilitates greater strength development.

Machines, on the other hand, keep the weight in only one trajectory so fewer muscles and motor units are recruited.

Since machines lock you into a fixed plane of movement, they reduce the contribution of the stabiliser muscles and so require less balance and skill to perform an exercise. This may be advantageous for beginners with poor motor skills, and poor muscle and postural awareness, but as muscles receive less stimulation so strength and size gains will be smaller.

Another problem with machines is that they do not accommodate the natural leverage of the body. Everyone has a unique set of levers, which will not exactly fit a machine. The resistance cams are set to match the strength curves of the 'average' person, which means that for everyone else the heaviest resistance occurs at inappropriate angles. A lower weight usually has to be selected in order to complete the movement correctly. Result: slower gains in strength and size.

Several different variations of the same exercise may be performed with free weights – e.g. bench presses with different grip widths or with the bench adjusted to different angles – thus making many different exercises possible. Machines offer fewer variations, thus potentially compromising overall development.

The case for machines

Machines and cables are good for isolating muscles and are generally safer than free weights, particularly when training without a partner or spotter: the weight stack can be returned to the starting position if you fail to complete a full repetition. Dumbbells and barbells can be dropped and plates can become unsecured.

Machines are good for beginners, for developing the basic motor skills and body awareness needed to control a movement. Once you have acquired this confidence, you can include more free-weight exercises in your routine.

WORKOUT ACCESSORIES

Training gloves

Training gloves give your palms just enough padding to improve your grip of the bar or dumbbells, and prevent calluses and blisters from forming on your hands. They are useful for any pressing, pulling or curling movement.

Using gloves is also more hygienic than using bare hands – weight training apparatus can be sweaty and dirty, and an ideal breeding place for germs.

Training belt

A training belt is thought to provide extra support for the lower back. However, it is only advantageous when using maximal weights, and then only for certain exercises performed vertically which place considerable stress on the vertebrae, such as heavy squats and dead lifts. It helps under these circumstances by increasing abdominal wall pressure. The tighter the belt, the greater the abdominal pressure against the spine, which thereby helps to protect the discs and other vulnerable structures. The abdominal wall should be drawn in towards the spine when lifting with a belt rather than being pushed out against it.

Do not use a belt for lighter exercises or if you have a lower-back injury or weakness. Using a belt for any other exercises in your workout can stimulate incorrect movement of the abdominal wall, leading to a weakening of the abdominal muscles.

Straps

Grip failure can be a limiting factor in pulling movements such as chins, seated rows and lat pull-downs. Up to a point, training without straps will help to develop the forearm muscles and strengthen your grip. However, once your grip strength starts to limit the amount of weight you can use or reduce the number of reps you can do, you should use straps. They will help you to focus on the muscle you are training and reduce the involvement of the limiting muscles. Straps are therefore advantageous for most back exercises and pulling movements performed with heavy weights.

Knee wraps

Knee wraps can help support the knee joint during heavy leg exercises such as dead lifts and squats because they assist the ligaments in stabilising the joint. As with training belts, do not rely on wraps if you have a knee injury or to help you lift heavier weights than your strength allows. They are best used for maximal weights (e.g. twice your body weight) rather than as a crutch for lighter sets.

SUMMARY OF KEY POINTS

- The benefits of training in a commercial gym include access to a wider range of equipment, professional instruction, greater motivation and social contact.
- A home gym offers greater privacy and convenience.
- Free weights develop better balance and coordination than machines, accommodate the natural leverage of the body and allow a more natural plane of movement, all facilitating greater strength development.
- Machines are safer and easier for beginners.
- Training gloves are useful for all weight trainers. Training belts should only be used for vertical exercises such as the squat when using maximal weights, and knee wraps for heavy leg exercises. Straps help to reduce the involvement of limiting muscles in certain pulling and back exercises.

GOAL-SETTING AND MOTIVATION

11

The key to success in any exercise programme is setting your goals and focusing your mind on reaching them. How well and how fast you achieve your goals depends on how motivated you are. But first you need to set clear goals and work out a plan to measure your success.

SMART GOALS

Goals should be SMART:
  S = specific
  M = measurable
  A = agreed
  R = realistic
  T = time scaled

Specific

Write down exactly what you want to achieve from your training programme. Avoid vague statements such as 'tone up' or 'get stronger' as these will not focus your mind on achieving a particular result. Your goals could include details of how much lean weight you wish to gain and how much fat you wish to lose. For example, 'lose 5 kg fat and gain 3 kg muscle'. You could also write down your desired body measurements, or how much weight you wish to lift on specific exercises such as the bench press, squat and dead lift.

To help you crystallise your goals, write down the reasons why you want to improve – whether it is increased muscle size, a more symmetrical physique, better sports performance or more energy. Go beyond the superficial reasons and find the inner motivations that are driving your goals. Research shows that it is the internal motivators that really drive us to success.

Measurable

You need to be able to measure your progress. Long-term goals can be broader in scope, but short-term goals must be quite specific. Indeed, the specific goals above could be in terms of your body weight, body fat measurements, girth measurements or the amount of weight lifted, which are clearly measurable too. For example, you may wish to set a goal of 60 kg for your maximal bench press, or reduce your body fat by 5 per cent. To help monitor your progress, photocopy the training log in Figure 11.1 to record the exact weight lifted, the number of repetitions and the number of sets completed at each workout, and use them to check what you have achieved each week against your long-term goal. Keep your training records for future reference as well. In the example given in Figure 11.2 for the bench press, 40/15 means 15 repetitions (reps) with 40 kg. (See also pp. 131–2.)

Agreed

Ideally, discuss and agree your goals with someone – a qualified instructor, your partner, or a friend. The most important thing is committing your goals to paper; this signals a commitment to

Figure 11.1 Training log

Exercise	Date		Date		Date		Date		Date		Date		Date	
	Set	(kg/reps)	Set	(kg/reps)	Set	(kg/reps)	Set	(kg/reps)	Set	(kg/reps)	Set	(kg/reps)	Set	(kg/reps)

Figure 11.2 Sample training log for a bench press					
	Date	**Date**	**Date**	**Date**	**Date**
	17/4	17/4	17/4	17/4	17/4
	Set	**Set**	**Set**	**Set**	**Set**
	1 (warm-up)	2	3	4	5*
Bench press	40 / 15	60 / 10	70 / 8	75 / 7	80 / 6

*Note: only advanced weight trainers should include five sets of any given exercise in their programme.

change. Write them in the form of a personal mission statement; then sign and date what you have written. Better still, ask someone else to sign the document as a witness, as you would with a contract. Then place a copy somewhere you can see it each day, such as on your desk or on a bulletin board. The goals will constantly remind you that they are waiting to be achieved. If you do not commit your goals to paper, then it is unlikely that you'll be able to commit to the work necessary to make them happen. Like a legal contract, this technique will keep your mind focused.

Realistic

The goals should be realistic – attainable for your body size, natural shape and lifestyle. There's nothing wrong with aiming for the top but, at the same time, be realistic. If it's a gold medal you seek, study the path others have taken to achieve that goal and check it against where you are starting from, and how much time and energy you have to follow a similar path.

Time scaled

Set a clear time scale for reaching your goals. Decide on a deadline – this prompts action and sets your plan in motion. Without a clear deadline, it's easy to put off starting your programme and you end up never achieving your goals.

Once you have fixed your major goals, set mini-goals, which can be reached in a relatively short period of time (such as 12 weeks), and long-term goals, which can be reached over, say, a year. You may even find it helpful to break up each 12-week goal into distinct segments and focus on the progress you make each week. For example, if your goal is to reduce your body fat percentage from 30 per cent to 20 per cent (see p. 201), break this down into smaller goals spread out over the course of several weeks. You could aim to achieve 24 per cent body fat within 12 weeks, but aim to reduce your body fat by 1 per cent every two weeks. Then aim to achieve 20 per cent within the next 12 weeks by reducing your body fat by 1 per cent every three weeks.

Set out a programme of activities or steps that you need to complete in order to reach each goal. These steps may include weight training three times a week, eating six balanced meals a day, and doing a cardio workout three times a week first thing in the morning. The key is to make sure each step is specific, realistic and achievable.

TIPS FOR SUCCESS

Visualise success

The ability to visualise success is one of the most effective tools of high-achievers. Use imagery to help you stick to your programme. Have a clear mental picture of how you will look or how you will perform at the end. Role models can help to motivate you. Pick one with a similar natural body type, shape and size as you – that way, you know you can achieve your goals and won't lose heart if you don't look similar to or perform like them after a period of training. You may find it helpful to cut out pictures from a magazine and keep these with your training log.

If you are finding it difficult to motivate yourself for a workout, visualise yourself successfully completing it. Use as many senses as possible – the sight of the gym, the sounds around you. See yourself loading the weights on the bar, see yourself completing each repetition, and hear the sound of voices or music in the gym.

Create a motivating environment

Training should give you a buzz and make you feel good about yourself. If you have to force yourself to work out when your heart is not in it, you will not train hard enough to make sufficient gains, and you are more likely to give up. So make sure you choose the right training environment (see also p. 125) and consider enlisting the help of a training partner (see below). That way, training will become a satisfying and empowering experience that you look forward to rather than dread.

Work out with a partner

Training with someone else will increase your motivation, make training more enjoyable, allow you to train harder, decrease the chances of you skipping workouts, and help you to stick to your training programme. Choose someone with similar goals to your own but not necessarily the same ability. The important thing is that you can motivate each other.

Measuring your body fat percentage

Skinfold testing and body fat monitors are the easiest and most accessible methods for estimating body fat.

- Skinfold callipers: calibrated callipers measure the layer of fat beneath the skin at a number of specific sites on the body, usually the biceps, triceps, below the shoulder blades and above the hip bone. The sum of the skinfolds is used in a simple equation to estimate your body fat percentage. The accuracy of this method depends almost entirely on the skill of the tester, as well as the precision of the callipers.
- Body fat monitor: this works on the principle of bioelectrical impedance. An electrode is placed on two specific points on the body – usually on one hand and the opposite foot – and an electric current is passed through them. Body fat creates an impedance, or resistance, to the current while fat-free mass permits a greater current flow. The body fat monitor measures the impedance and then uses additional information you've provided (such as your sex and height) to calculate your percentage of fat-free mass and the percentage of body fat. The accuracy depends on hydration, skin temperature, and alcohol and food consumption. It is less accurate for very lean or obese individuals.

Monitor your progress

Keep a training and nutrition diary to record your progress. Remember, achieving your goals will not happen overnight. It comes after weeks or months of committed effort. Monitor your progress on a regular basis so you can check that your actions are producing the results you want. If they are not, you need to take the necessary steps to get you back on track. Training and nutrition diaries can be great motivators during workouts. Look back over your notes at the end

Table 11.1	Measurement log						
	Date	**Chest**	**Waist**	**Hips**	**Thigh**	**Arm**	**Body fat %**
Start							
Week 1							
Week 2							
Week 3							
Week 4							
Week 5							
Week 6							
Week 7							
Week 8							
Week 9							
Week 10							
Week 11							
Week 12							

of each week. If your performance matches your goals, reward yourself.

Buy a notebook so that you can record the following details:

- details of each exercise, sets, reps and how much weight you used (using an exercise log like that in Figure 11.1)
- how you felt before and after each workout
- what and how much you ate each day
- details of any other exercise you took
- your body measurements, including percentage body fat (see 'Measuring your body fat percentage' in the accompanying box), waist, chest, hip, leg and arm circumference measurements, or just how snugly your clothes fit (see the 'Measurement log' in Table 11.1; you may wish to photocopy this or redraw it so that you can fill in your details).

Photographs taken before you start your new programme and then at intervals throughout your training will help to give you feedback on your progress. This is more objective than simply looking in the mirror.

Vary your workouts

Your body adapts to a certain workload and soon stops developing. Change your workout periodically to keep your body challenged and to keep boredom at bay. When you start a strength training programme, gains are rapid but then slow down or reach a plateau. Ask your gym instructor to review or devise a more intense workout when you get in a rut. Try changing the following aspects of your programme (see also Chapter 13):

- the exercises for each body part
- the split of your programme
- the order of exercises
- the weights used.

Also take a complete rest from weight training every few months and spend a week or two doing a completely different activity.

Use a personal trainer

If you do not have a training partner or you need extra motivation, consider using a personal trainer either on an occasional or regular basis. A personal trainer will not only design your programme but will help keep you motivated. They will make sure that you are on track with your goals and that you don't skip any workouts, give you advice on a whole range of subjects, help you get more out of your training, and also allow you to train at a time that is convenient for you.

To find a personal trainer ask friends for recommendations or check with your gym for trainers who are qualified to NVQ Level 3 and have a qualification in personal training. Also check out their references and make sure that they are insured. The Exercise Register (www.exercise register.com) lists fully qualified and insured trainers in the UK.

Reward yourself

Give yourself rewards when you have reached a goal, no matter how small. This could be something as simple as a star for reaching your weekly target, or a new training outfit, a trip to the theatre, a meal out, new clothes or a sports massage appointment for reaching the bigger goals.

SUMMARY OF KEY POINTS

- It is imperative to set clear short-term and long-term goals before you embark on any fitness programme.
- Goals should be SMART: specific, measurable, agreed, realistic and time scaled.
- Motivation can be increased by visualisation techniques, training with a partner, keeping a training log and a record of your measurements, varying your routine, using a personal trainer, and rewarding your progress.

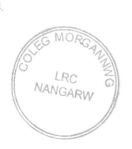

TRAINING PRINCIPLES AND METHODS

12

Gaining a greater understanding of training principles and methods will help you target your training programme more effectively.

PROGRESSIVE RESISTANCE TRAINING

Progressive resistance (or 'overload' training) is a calculated method of progressively working your muscles harder and harder to induce gains in strength, mass or endurance. When you train with heavy weights, they adapt by getting stronger and stronger.

As you become stronger, fewer motor units (and therefore fewer muscle fibres) are needed to perform the same exercise – your muscles become more efficient at performing particular movements – so you have to subject your muscles to progressive amounts of overload. If you were to stick to the same workout – the same exercises, weights, sets, rep schemes and rep speeds – your muscles would stop adapting and growing, and you would only maintain your strength.

Sets and reps

The basic unit of weight training is the repetition ('rep'). A repetition is one complete movement in the exercise, from the starting position to a position of maximum contraction and then back to the starting position. This ensures that you complete what is called the full range of move-ment (ROM). On the bench press, for example, lowering the bar to your chest (the eccentric, or negative, part of the rep) and pushing it back up from your chest (the concentric, or positive, part of the rep) is one repetition.

These repetitions are grouped together in sets. If you perform 10 repetitions of the bench press before taking a rest, those 10 repetitions constitute a set.

Training to failure

When training to failure, you perform repetitions until you can no longer lift the weight through the concentric (or positive) part of the movement using proper form. Each exercise has a 'sticking point' during the concentric phase – the part of the movement where gravity and unfavourable leverage make it hardest, and this is usually the

> ### One-rep max
>
> One-rep max (1RM) is the heaviest weight that you can lift for one – and just one – repetition. In other words, you can do a maximum of one repetition only for a given weight. This can be calculated either directly (by performing your 1RM after a thorough warm-up) or indirectly by performing a 3RM (which is safer), then extrapolating this to what your 1RM should be. Alternatively, find a weight with which you can just perform six repetitions. This is equivalent to approximately 70–80 per cent of your 1RM.

part of the movement at which the point of muscular failure is reached. Training to the point of failure allows you to recruit the largest number of motor units, which in turn results in maximal muscle-fibre stimulation.

TRAINING TECHNIQUE

Training with proper form is crucial to avoid injury and maximise results. Your muscles don't know how much weight is on the bar but they do respond to the magnitude of tension developed during each movement. High levels of tension are achieved with proper form and relatively heavy weights. Many weight trainers get into the habit of using poor training form in order to lift more weight or squeeze out a couple of extra repetitions, but that does not produce better results. If you are unsure of an exercise, get assistance from an instructor or personal trainer, who will be able to reinforce good technique. Pay close attention to the descriptions for each exercise in Part Two of this book and the following technique tips.

1. Always warm up properly before starting your workout. Never train a cold muscle as this increases injury risk.
2. Select a suitable weight that will allow you to complete the desired number of repetitions safely. Do not be tempted to lift heavier weights before you have developed sufficient strength in your muscles, tendons and ligaments.
3. The general rule of thumb is to breathe out on the concentric (or positive) part of the movement (when you lift the weight) and breathe in on the eccentric (or negative) part of the movement (lowering the weight). Never hold your breath.
4. Perform each repetition using the complete ROM, taking the muscle from its fully

extended position to its fully contracted position. Partial repetitions will develop strength only in that portion of the movement, and produce only slow overall gains. Also avoid cheating movements as these will reduce the training stimulus and increase injury risk.

5. Maintain full control of the weight throughout the movement. Swinging a weight too fast means momentum takes over to bear the load rather than the target muscles, putting your joints at risk of injury.
6. Focus on both the concentric and eccentric phases of each movement. Resist the weight as you return it slowly to the starting position.
7. To find the correct training tempo, count to two as you lift the weight, and count to three as you lower the weight. Hold the fully contracted position for a count of one (but do not relax) before returning the weight to the starting position.
8. Visualising your target muscle contracting and relaxing will not only help you perform the exercise with good technique but will also help you do more repetitions. For example, as you press the bar up for a bench press, visualise your chest muscles contracting and getting stronger. This strategy reinforces the powerful mind–body link, which gives you more control over your body and, ultimately, greater physical gains.
9. Ideally, stretch the target muscles between sets, holding each stretch for a minimum of 8 seconds.
10. Perform longer (developmental) stretches immediately after the workout. Each stretch should be held for 30–60 seconds.

Pyramid training

Pyramid training is a form of multiple-set training in which the weight is increased in each set and the number of repetitions reduced. This allows you to warm up a muscle group gradually, and prepare it over the course of a few sets to cope with heavier weights by the end of the sets – hence allowing the muscles to achieve greater overload, and allowing you to develop greater size and strength. A typical pyramid is shown in Figure 12.1. Select a weight that will enable you to reach near or complete failure at the end of each set.

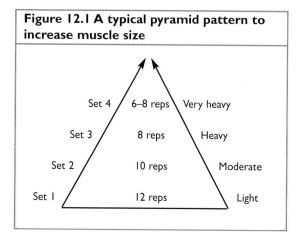

Figure 12.1 A typical pyramid pattern to increase muscle size

Set 4 / 6–8 reps \ Very heavy

Set 3 / 8 reps \ Heavy

Set 2 / 10 reps \ Moderate

Set 1 / 12 reps \ Light

Eccentric training (negatives)

In eccentric training, a spotter assists you in lifting the bar (the concentric phase), and then you control the weight on the eccentric (lowering) phase. This technique allows you to use a heavier weight (110–160 per cent 1RM) so should be performed after a thorough warm-up and particularly at the end of a set after you have reached muscular failure. Focus on lowering the weight very slowly.

The principle behind this technique is that it produces greater muscle growth than conventional (concentric) training techniques.[1,2] During an eccentric contraction there is more mechanical load per motor unit. As a result, eccentric training can generate up to two-thirds more tension in the muscle than concentric training. Increased tension provides a greater stimulus to the muscle fibres, which, in turn, means greater strength and growth.

As this is a very intense training method, limit eccentric training to one exercise per muscle group in any one workout, performing it at the end of only one or two sets. You will need to allow longer rest intervals between sets, and following hard eccentric training you will experience greater muscle soreness because of the greater resulting muscle fibre damage. Recovery may take up to 10 days, so you should allow at least 10–14 days between muscle group workouts employing this technique. For example, if you perform eccentric training on the chest on Monday, do not use it for the chest again for two weeks.

Forced, or assisted, rep training

With forced rep training you enlist the help of a spotter so that you can continue past the point of failure and therefore complete a couple of extra repetitions. The spotter should give just enough support to keep the weight moving through the sticking point.

You should only use this training technique for the last one or two reps of your heaviest sets, and should be able to complete at least six reps on your own in the correct form before the spotter assists you. If you cannot complete six reps, reduce the weight.

The advantage of forced rep training is that you can work past the point of muscular failure and thus increase the overload. For example, if you can normally complete six reps at 70 kg on the bench press, the forced rep training method may enable you to complete eight reps, thus increasing the amount of stress that your pectorals receive. Whether this ultimately results in greater muscle hypertrophy, however, is a controversial issue.

Forced reps should only be used during intense training cycles and you should limit this method to once a week per muscle group.

Descending (drop) sets

This method is particularly useful for reaching overload if you are training without a partner or spotter and cannot use eccentric or forced rep training.

With descending sets you complete as many repetitions in strict form as you can, then – without resting – you reduce the weight by 20–50 per cent and continue performing repetitions (usually four to six) until you reach the point of failure again. Repeat this process if you wish.

Again, the objective is to stimulate as many motor units as possible. The first reps, performed with a heavy weight, stimulate the FT muscle fibres; subsequent reps performed with lighter weights stimulate mainly ST fibres. So this method allows you to train for strength, muscle size and endurance within the same set.

This method is safest for exercises with dumbbells and machines since you need to be able to return the weight safely and quickly when your muscles have reached failure. Examples of suitable exercises include: leg extensions, leg curls, dumbbell presses, flyes, lateral raises, dumbbell biceps curls, lat pull-downs, seated rows and triceps push-downs. For example, if you are performing a set of lateral raises with 10 kg dumbbells, complete as many reps as you can in strict form – say, eight. Return the dumbbells to the floor, pick up a pair of 7.5 kg dumbbells and perform as many as you can until you reach failure – say, five. Repeat with 5 kg dumbbells.

Since this method is very fatiguing, it should only be used for selected exercises and only for the last one or two sets, providing maximum stimulation to the muscle when it is fatigued. You will need to leave slightly longer rest intervals between descending sets (say two to three min-

utes) and reduce the total number of sets per muscle group. Again, use this method sparingly, once every three weeks.

Superset training

This involves performing two or more exercises for a given body part in a row, and there are two methods, as described below.

SUPERSETS FOR THE SAME MUSCLE GROUPS

This method involves two or more exercises for the same muscle group – for example, dumbbell shoulder press followed by lateral raises and upright rows for the shoulders. The advantage is that the stress on the muscle is increased as the muscle can be worked from slightly different angles, thus involving more muscle fibres. It also increases the blood flow to the muscle due to the increased energy demand, providing greater stimulation for hypertrophy. However, this type of superset training should not be used for every body part or at every workout as it is very intense and may lead to overtraining.

SUPERSETS FOR OPPOSING MUSCLE GROUPS

This less intense method involves performing two exercises for opposing muscle groups – for example, biceps curls followed by triceps extensions, or leg extensions followed by leg curls. The advantage of this method is that the blood is kept within the same area of the body, thus encouraging a greater flow and bringing more fuel, oxygen and nutrients to the muscle. Since the rest period is eliminated, it is also a good way of reducing your workout time, particularly useful if you have only a limited period in which to train.

Unlike supersetting the same muscle group, this method does not significantly increase the muscle overload. However, it does increase the demands on your cardiovascular system since the rest periods are greatly reduced, and can therefore help to improve lactic acid tolerance, raise the anaerobic threshold and develop better stamina.

Following each superset you should take a two- to three-minute rest.

Pre-exhaustion training

With pre-exhaustion training the larger muscle (prime mover) is partially exhausted by performing an isolation exercise prior to performing the compound exercise. For example, performing flyes before bench presses pre-exhausts the pectorals so that when you perform the bench presses, your pectorals will fatigue before, or at the same time as, the triceps and front deltoids. (You will probably need to reduce the weight you use for the bench presses.) There is no need to change the rest intervals between sets. The objective is to change the usual recruitment pattern of the muscle fibres involved and enable you to stimulate more muscle.

Like other advanced training methods, pre-exhaustion training should only be used for selected exercises and you should limit this method to once a week per muscle group.

Getting pumped

The 'pump' that you get during heavy training is not the same as muscle growth. This temporary increase in muscle size is largely the result of water accumulating inside the muscle fibres making the muscle look larger. The majority of this water returns to the blood a few hours after training and so the pump disappears.

CORE TRAINING

The benefits

Core training is based on the idea that by training the muscles surrounding the torso, pelvis and spine, you can increase stability throughout your entire body. Training your 'core' – hips/torso/mid-section – helps builds better balance and posture by aligning your body correctly. It also helps improve performance and prevent injury. It will help strengthen a weak lower back, for example, or tone a flabby mid-section. When you work to strengthen and stabilise your core, you strengthen your body's power base.

How to do it

There are many exercises that challenge core stability; Pilates is one of the best-known stability programmes. Others involve exercising from an unstable base such as a wobble board or exercise ball, which places a higher demand on the deep muscles in the core – or trunk – as well as on your motor control system because you constantly have to stabilise yourself as the ball or board rolls around. It also changes the way your neuromuscular system coordinates movement as you're using your legs to hold you up, and your abdominals and back to keep your whole body stable. Traditional exercises have little effect on core stability as they do not work the trunk stabilisers – the transverse abdominis (TVA) and the lumbar multifidus – but doing exercises on a ball or wobble board challenges stability on many planes of movement, so works these muscles more effectively.

The basics

The first step in core training is to find your neutral posture, where your joints are aligned correctly to each other. To locate this, follow the steps outlined below.

- Stand with your feet hip-width apart, knees relaxed.
- Let your shoulders drop down and away from your ears.
- Lengthen your spine and neck – imagine a string, attached to the top of your head, pulling you up to the ceiling.
- Contract your abdominal muscles, drawing the navel in towards your spine.
- Adjust the tilt of your pelvis so that it is in a neutral position. You should be able to draw a line vertically from your shoulders to your hips to your feet.

Core training with weights

Once you have mastered maintaining your neutral posture, you'll be training your core muscles during any activity. Try to integrate core training into your weights workouts. Maintain constant tension in your abdominals and keep your spine in neutral alignment at all times.

Seated exercises, such as shoulder presses or biceps curl, can be performed on an exercise ball. Hold in your abdominals and keep your back in the neutral posture – your shoulders and hips should form a straight line. Try using an exercise ball instead of a bench for doing lying dumbbell presses and flyes. Not only will you target your chest but you'll also be working your core muscles to maintain balance and stability on the ball. You will need to use lighter weights than usual.

SUMMARY OF KEY POINTS

- Set training and pyramid training form the core of any training programme for strength, power or size.
- Advanced training methods – such as eccentric training, forced rep training, descending sets, supersets and pre-exhaustion – allow you to train with greater intensity and experience continued gains.
- Core training can be integrated into weights workouts to improve balance, posture and performance, prevent injury and strengthen the lower back.

DESIGNING A PROGRAMME

Understanding the components of a training programme will help you to work out more effectively and achieve your goals. A training programme contains several key variables, which you can manipulate to meet your goals.[1,2,3]

SELECTION OF EXERCISES

The exercises you select for your programme should result in equal stimulation of each muscle group, and ensure that no muscle group is left out.

Keep your muscles growing by having a greater repertoire of exercises from which to choose. You can do this by frequently changing the exercises you perform for each muscle group and by using variations of standard exercises in different body positions to emphasise different parts of the muscle group.

Compound vs isolation exercises

Compound, or multi-joint, exercises cause greatest stimulation of the muscle fibres and should form the basis of strength- and mass-building programmes. They involve one or more large muscle groups (i.e. the chest, legs, shoulders, back, hips) and work across two or more major joints. For example, the bench press is a compound exercise that is used primarily to target the pectoral muscles but also involves the triceps and front deltoids. Therefore, the exercise stimulates three muscle groups. It is a multi-joint exercise because the movement involves both arm flexion (the shoulder joint) and extension of the forearm (the elbow joint).

Isolation, or single-joint, exercises involve smaller muscle groups (i.e. biceps, triceps, brachioradialis, erector spinae) and only one main joint. For example, the dumbbell flye is an isolation exercise that is used primarily to target the pectorals. The elbows are kept at a fixed angle throughout the ROM and so no other muscle groups are worked. It is a single-joint exercise as it only works around the shoulder joint.

Isolation exercises are often included in beginner programmes because they are easier to learn and execute using good form. Once you have mastered the basic movement patterns, plan your programme around compound exercises that stimulate a greater number of muscle fibres.

ORDER OF EXERCISES

The order in which you perform your exercises will affect the energy and effort you are able to put into the next exercise. For example, performing two consecutive exercises that both stimulate the same muscle group reduces the effort you can put into the second one. The order can be changed according to the aspect of strength you wish to develop, and there are four methods, as outlined below.

1. Largest to smallest

The most usual way of ordering exercises is to work from the largest muscle groups to the smallest. Therefore, compound exercises that stimulate the largest muscle groups are performed first in your workout, followed by the isolation exercises. This is because the compound exercises require the most effort and concentration, and are very difficult to perform correctly and safely if your muscles are fatigued. For example, in a leg workout you would perform compound exercises such as squats and leg presses before isolation exercises such as leg extensions and leg curls.

Advanced trainers sometimes reverse this order so as to break through a training plateau. This is called pre-exhaustion and involves deliberately fatiguing a large muscle group by performing isolation exercises before the compound exercise (see p. 140).

2. Alternating upper- and lower-body circuit

Alternating upper- and lower-body exercises is particularly suitable for beginners who would otherwise find performing several exercises for one area in one go too demanding. This method allows each muscle group to recover more fully between exercises, and is also good for people with limited training time available because it minimises rest intervals – you can perform an upper-body exercise straight after a lower-body exercise without resting. Because rest periods are minimised, you also get a greater cardiovascular effect compared with more conventional strength training programmes. On the downside, this method generally results in less stimulation of each muscle group, and can result in slower strength and mass gains. Therefore, it would be less suitable for advanced weight trainers.

3. Alternating 'push' and 'pull' exercises

Alternating pushing exercises (e.g. bench press) and pulling exercises (e.g. seated row) is also suitable for beginners, those resuming strength training and those with limited training time available. As with alternating upper- and lower-body exercises, this method is a very good way of reducing your rest periods because, while you are performing a pulling exercise (the seated row), the opposing muscle group used in the pushing exercise (the bench press) is recovering. You will not need to rest, yet you can still use maximum effort for each set. If you were to arrange several pushing exercises together (e.g. bench press, shoulder press, triceps extensions), you might have to reduce the amount of weight or number of repetitions used because the triceps (a muscle used in all three exercises) will become fatigued.

4. Supersets

This training method involves two or more sets of different exercises performed consecutively with no rest period between. As it is very demanding, supersets are best suited to advanced weight trainers (see pp. 172–5).

SETS AND REPS

The number of sets and reps you perform depends on your goals, training experience, the number of muscle groups trained per session and the size of the muscle group being trained. Table 13.1 gives guidelines for the number of sets and repetitions, weight and rest intervals commonly prescribed for strength, power, hypertrophy and muscular endurance training programmes.

Table 13.1	Sets, repetitions, weight and rest interval guidelines for different training goals				
Training goal	Number of sets per exercise	Number of repetitions	Weight (% 1RM)	Rest interval	Training tempo*
Maximum strength	2–6	< 6	Heavy (> 85)	2–5 min	1:2
Power	3–5	1–5	Heavy (75–85)	2–5 min	Explosive: 1
Muscle size	3–6	6–12	67–85	30–90 s	2:3
Muscular endurance	2–3	> 12	Low (< 67)	< 30 s	2:3

*The training tempo is the number of counts for the concentric (lifting) action, followed by the number of counts for the eccentric (lowering) action, e.g. 2:3 is 2 counts concentric, 3 counts eccentric.

Maximum strength

Maximum strength is developed using heavy weights and low-repetition sets. The consensus guideline is to perform two to six sets of six or fewer repetitions for the compound exercises.[1,3,4] Only one to three sets are necessary for isolation exercises.[5] Clearly you should select a weight that causes you to use maximum effort for that set – that is, reach the point of failure on the last repetition (between 85–100 per cent 1RM). Your rest intervals between sets should be three to four minutes to allow sufficient recovery. Maximum strength workouts are centred on the compound exercises such as squats, bench presses and shoulder presses.

Power

Performing an exercise very quickly or explosively develops power. It can be developed with plyometrics and speed drills, as well as weightlifting exercises. For example, squat jumps and alternate leg bounding (plyometrics), 40 m dashes, shuttle runs (speed drills), power cleans, power pulls or any compound weight training exercises (e.g. leg press, squat) performed explosively would all be suitable methods of developing neuromuscular activity and power. Power exercises would be suitable for intermediate and advanced weight trainers, Olympic lifters and athletes who use power movements in their particular sport. For example, basketball, football, sprinting and most field athletic events (such as the high jump and long jump) involve explosive activities, so power training would benefit your performance.

However, only experienced lifters and athletes should use this type of training as it could be dangerous if attempted using imperfect technique. It is important that the weight is kept under good control even when it is moved rapidly. The consensus guideline is three to five sets of one to five repetitions,[1,6] using moderate (75–85 per cent 1RM), rather than maximal weights. Slightly lighter weights allow you to perform the exercise with maximum speed and therefore generate the greatest power output: output almost doubles when reducing the weight from 100 per cent 1RM to 90 per cent 1RM.[7]

Muscle size

Training for muscle size (hypertrophy) requires a higher training volume compared with pure strength and power training – in other words, more repetitions, sets and a greater cumulative amount of weight lifted per workout. The consensus guideline is a moderate number of repetitions (6–12) and three to six sets per exercise performed with a moderate to heavy weight (67–85 per cent 1RM) and short to moderate rest intervals (30–90 seconds).[1,3,8]

You can expect parallel increases in both muscle size and strength with this type of training programme. For overall size development, your programme should be based around compound exercises that stimulate the large muscle groups (e.g. squats, bench presses, shoulder presses, lat pull-downs). More advanced weight trainers and bodybuilders use two to four exercises per muscle group, including at least one or two compound exercises. They use a split training system (see below), allowing them to train with high intensity.

Muscular endurance

Muscular endurance is the ability of a muscle or muscle group to sustain sub-maximal force over a period of time. This type of training increases the aerobic capacity of the muscles rather than muscle size and strength, and is developed by using a higher number of repetitions (12 or more) per set and minimal rest intervals between sets – typically less than 30 seconds.[1,3] The weights lifted are lighter and fewer sets are performed per muscle group, usually two or three. Therefore, the intensity is very low and the overall volume high.

This type of workout is suitable for beginners but also for advanced weight trainers wishing to improve this aspect of their fitness. Most circuit weight training programmes, which alternate upper- and lower-body exercises or opposing

How fast should you lift?

Perhaps the most important principle for stimulating muscle growth is the time that the muscle is under tension – i.e. the time your muscles are actually working. For example, if you blast a set of 10 repetitions as fast as possible, your total time under tension will be just a few seconds. This is not sufficient to cause your muscles to grow, regardless of the amount of weight you lift.

Typically, the time under tension should be 30–70 seconds. Anything more or less would be counterproductive and result in very little gain.

The way to achieve the correct set duration is to adjust your training tempo. For example, if you are working in relatively low-rep ranges (say, 6–8), you will have to adjust your training tempo – particularly on the eccentric (lowering) part of the movement – in order for that set's time under tension to reach at least 30 seconds. If you are working in a higher-rep range (say, 10–12), the training tempo should be a little quicker so that you won't exceed the 30–70 seconds' time under tension range.

muscle groups and limit rest intervals to 30 seconds or less, would promote muscular endurance.

Full-body routine vs split workouts

If you plan to train all major muscle groups in your workout (a full-body routine), you should perform one or two sets of each exercise and only one or two exercises per muscle group, making a total of 15–20 sets.

As you progress to a split routine, dividing your whole-body workout into two or three separate workouts, you will be able to perform more sets per muscle group. The larger muscle groups (legs, back, chest, shoulders) generally require more sets (e.g. 6–12) than the smaller muscle groups (biceps, triceps), which require fewer sets (e.g. 3–8) for the advanced weight trainer to achieve sufficient stimulation.

TRAINING INTENSITY

Training intensity serves as the major stimulus for muscle growth. By increasing your training intensity, you provide a bigger stimulus for muscle growth. You can increase the intensity by increasing the amount of weight, number of sets or repetitions, and the number of exercises, or reducing rest intervals between sets. The exact combination you choose depends on your goals, strength, power, size or muscular endurance.

REST PERIODS BETWEEN WORKOUTS

Rest between workouts is as important as the training itself. This is when replenishment, recovery, adaptation and growth take place. Let's take a look at what happens.

During and immediately after a workout your body is in a catabolic state (i.e. breaking down proteins) and levels of stress hormones such as cortisol are high. As you start to recover from your workout, levels of muscle-promoting hormones such as testosterone gradually rise, the damaged muscle proteins are replaced with new muscle proteins and glycogen stores are also restored (see pp. 24–5). Clearly, these processes take time. It is only after completion of the recovery process that the muscles can grow and strengthen. If you attempt to train your muscles before the process is complete then you will experience only minimal growth or none at all. In other words, training before you have recovered fully is counterproductive.

The rest period you need to leave between workouts depends on the intensity and duration of your workout, your training experience and your diet.

Training intensity and duration

The more intense your workout, the longer the recovery time required before your next training session. There is no easy or accurate way of predicting your recovery time between workouts. In the laboratory, scientists can measure the blood levels of muscle metabolites such as 3-methyl histidine and creatine phosphokinase, but this is clearly not a practical solution for everyday training. Instead, a certain amount of guesswork is required as you have to judge the 'feel' of your muscles. When your muscles have regained their pre-workout capacity – measured by testing your strength – you have probably recovered. Obviously, if your muscles still feel sore, stiff or weak, then they have not recovered. If you find yourself stronger and able to work out harder, then you know your muscles have recovered fully.

In general, upper-body muscles can recover more quickly from heavy workouts than lower-body muscles. Also, it takes longer to recover from compound exercises than isolation exercises.

Training experience

The American College of Sports Medicine recommends that beginners train two or three times a week on non-consecutive days. As you become more experienced and better conditioned, you can increase your workout frequency to four or more times a week.

As a general guideline, beginners should leave a minimum of one day and a maximum of three days' recovery between workouts. Experienced weight trainers will need to leave three to seven days between training the same muscle group due to the greater workout intensity. However, you can train four or more times a week by using a split routine – that is, dividing your major muscle groups into two or more separate workouts (see p. 143). That way, you can still allow a minimum of three days' rest between training each muscle group.

Your diet

During recovery, your muscle glycogen stores are replenished and muscle tissue repaired. The time it takes to replenish muscle glycogen depends on the severity of depletion, and the amount and timing of carbohydrate intake in your diet. On average, this takes between 24 hours and three days. You also need to ensure you consume enough protein to provide the raw material for new muscle growth. An inadequate intake will result in slower repair and growth, and so your strength gains will be compromised. On the other hand, an excessive intake will not further enhance muscle growth or strength. For more detail on diet, see Part One.

SUMMARY OF KEY POINTS

- The main components of a programme are the selection of exercises, ordering of exercises, amount of sets and reps, rest periods, and the training intensity.

- The exercises you select for your workout depend on your specific goals and your level of experience. For strength, mass and endurance, select maximum-stimulation exercises.
- The ordering of your exercises affects the energy and effort you are able to put into the next exercise. Going from the largest to the smallest muscle groups is recommended for beginners and advanced weight trainers, while performing supersets for the same muscle group is recommended only for advanced weight trainers.
- The number of sets you perform depends on the size of the muscle group being trained, the number of muscle groups trained per session and your training experience.
- The rest period you need to leave between workouts depends on the intensity and duration of your workout, your training experience, and your diet.
- You can increase your training and intensity by increasing the amount of weight, number of sets or repetitions, number of exercises, or reducing rest intervals between sets.
- Maximum strength is developed using heavy weights and low-repetition sets, typically two to six sets of six or fewer repetitions.
- Power is developed by performing a compound exercise explosively – typically five sets of one to five repetitions using moderate weights (75–85 per cent 1RM).
- Muscle size (hypertrophy) is best developed using moderate to heavy weights (67–85 per cent 1RM) and moderate repetition sets, typically 6–12 repetitions for three to six sets.
- Muscular endurance is developed by using lighter weights, higher repetitions (12 or more) and minimal rest intervals (typically less than 30 seconds).

WARMING UP

WHY WARM UP?

It is important to warm up before beginning your workout because:
• it helps reduce the chances of injury
• it can improve your performance.
Muscles respond better to exercise if they are properly prepared for the coming workload. Warming up increases blood flow to the muscles and lubricates the joints because the fluid surrounding them becomes less viscous so the joint can move more smoothly and efficiently. At rest, muscles receive only about 15 per cent of your total blood supply, but during exercise the requirement for fuel and oxygen increases sharply and they may need up to 80 per cent of the total blood flow to meet the demand. Obviously, it takes time to re-route the blood, and this cannot be achieved efficiently if you omit the warm-up and start exercising vigorously.

Warming up also improves the elasticity of the muscles, enabling them to work harder, more efficiently and for longer before they fatigue, as well as allowing nerve impulses to be transmitted faster.

Importantly, warming up also prepares you mentally for the work ahead; it increases your arousal level and motivation. Performing one or two warm-up sets with light weights acts as a mental rehearsal and means that you can perform your subsequent heavier sets more effectively.

HOW TO DO IT

The time taken on this part of your workout depends to a large extent on the temperature of your surroundings – the cooler the environment, the longer it will take to raise your body temperature. Your warm-up should include the following three components.

1. Light cardiovascular work (5–10 minutes) to raise your body temperature and prepare your body for more strenuous exercise. This can be done on a stationary bike, treadmill, stepper, rower or elliptical trainer. Make sure you exercise continuously for at least five minutes at an intensity that allows you to break a sweat.

2. Mobilisation of the major joints – this could include movements such as arm circles, knee bends and shoulder circles, which take the joints through their full ROM. These are not stretching exercises as they are continuous and do not increase the ROM.

3. Warm-up sets with light weights and high repetitions. Never embark on your working (heavy) sets straightaway because your muscles won't be properly warmed up and you will risk injury. Start with one or two sets using very light weights – around 25–50 per cent 1RM (see p. 134) – for 15–20 repetitions to warm up the target muscles, ligaments and joints, and to rehearse the action to be performed.

TO STRETCH OR NOT TO STRETCH?

Previously it was thought that stretching before strenuous activity would help prepare the muscles for exercise and reduce the risk of injury. However, more recent research suggests that stretching before you start training is unlikely to benefit your performance and, ironically, may even reduce your strength and increase the risk of injury.[1,2,3]

There is no evidence either that pre-exercise stretching prevents post-exercise soreness or tenderness. Most experts believe that stretching is best kept to a minimum prior to strength and power training. An active warm-up, including the three components outlined above, is more effective.

STRETCHING

15

Most people imagine gym-goers to be muscle-bound, and lacking in mobility and graceful posture. Indeed, many bodybuilders who neglect to stretch do fit that image. Stretching is highly beneficial for anyone involved in strength training. Not only does it provide numerous health benefits but it can also enhance your muscle size and shape.

This chapter gives you a thorough checklist on safe and effective stretching, and explains exactly what happens in your muscles when you stretch. Finally, it gives you a step-by-step guide to the essential stretches that will benefit your workouts.

WHY STRETCH?

The benefits of a good stretching programme include:
- reduced risk of muscle strain, joint injuries and back problems
- reduced post-exercise muscle soreness
- speedier recovery
- increased ROM and coordination
- greater strength gains due to greater ROM
- improved body awareness
- better physical and mental relaxation.

HOW CAN STRETCHING HELP ENHANCE MUSCLE SIZE AND SHAPE?

Incorporating key stretches into your strength training programme will result in greater muscle growth and the enhancement of muscle shape. Failing to stretch will not only limit your ROM but also your growth rate.

Stretching elongates the fascia, a strong protective sheath of connective tissue covering all muscles and their cells, allowing the muscle underneath room in which to grow. Fascia tissue can become thick and tough if the muscles are not stretched and are subjected to a limited ROM. The best time to stretch the fascia is when the muscles are very warm and 'pumped' (i.e. full of blood, see p. 136). This occurs during and after a workout, so stretch between and after sets, and at the end of your training session.

Stretching increases flexibility, giving the muscles and joints a greater ROM. It can prevent muscle soreness and promote faster recovery between workouts, helping to release lactic acid from the muscle cells into the bloodstream so that it does not hinder further muscle contraction. Therefore, stretching during your workout may enable you to train harder and longer.

Stretching improves posture as well, and gives the body a more athletic or graceful appearance instead of that clumsy awkward gait that many bodybuilders develop.

HOW DO MUSCLES STRETCH?

The muscles contain receptors called muscle spindles, which register information about the muscle's length and rate of change of length. One of their main jobs is to protect the muscles from injury. So whenever there is a rapid change in muscle length, a reflex action is set up to shorten or contract it instead.

Tendons – which attach muscles to bone – also contain receptors called golgi tendon organs (GTOs), registering information about the degree of tension in the tendon. When a high force is registered, the GTOs enable the muscle to relax in an attempt to reduce the tension, thus acting as a safety mechanism. If the intensity of a muscular contraction or stretch exceeds a certain critical point, an immediate reflex occurs to inhibit the contraction or stretch. As a result, the muscle instantly relaxes and the excessive tension is removed, and with it the possibility of injury. In other words, the GTOs shut down the muscle to prevent injury. If the GTOs did not exist, it would be possible to have a stretch or contraction so powerful that the muscle or tendon would be torn from its attachments!

Bouncing, uncontrolled or forced movements cause the greatest reflex response. Thus ballistic stretching can cause the muscle to contract and so increase the chance of injury. Static stretching that is carried out slowly and in a controlled manner will lead to a reflex relaxation of the muscle.

Strength through stretching is related to your GTO threshold, which limits a contraction well short of the point at which tendons would be injured. Stretching gives the muscles the ability to contract more efficiently without shutting down in response to stretched tendons. Obviously, it is desirable to have a high GTO reflex threshold, as this allows you to handle heavier weights and do more reps without the GTOs inhibiting muscle action. The higher the GTO threshold, the more intensely you can train, and the greater the gains in size and strength. Stretching your muscles regularly can help raise your GTO threshold, some experts estimate, by up to 15–20 per cent.

HOW TO PERFORM STRETCHES

You should only stretch when your body is warm and the muscle is receiving an increased blood flow. Stretching a cold muscle increases the risk of injury and reduces the effectiveness of the stretch. Here are some basic guidelines.

1. Ideally, stretching should be done after a workout and also between sets.
2. Alternatively, stretch between workouts as a separate session, but only after a thorough warm-up (5–10 minutes of some light aerobic activity or a hot bath).
3. Perform static stretches and avoid bouncing. This is a far safer method of stretching a muscle.
4. Gradually ease into position, all the time focusing on relaxing the muscle.
5. Stretch only as far as is comfortable and then hold that position. As the muscle relaxes, ease further into the stretch, gradually increasing the ROM.
6. Never hold your breath. Exhale and relax as you go into the stretch and then breathe normally.
7. Never go past the point of discomfort or pain. You could pull or tear the muscle/tendon.
8. Stretches performed at the end of a workout, or during a separate session (developmental stretching), should be held for 30 seconds or more to allow stretching in the connective tissue and muscle.
9. Release from the stretch slowly.

THE STRETCHES

Standing quadriceps stretch

- Hold on to a sturdy support.
- Bend one leg behind you and hold the ankle.
- Keep your thighs level, knees close, keep a small gap between your heel and backside, and push your hips forwards until you feel a good stretch.
- Repeat on the other side.

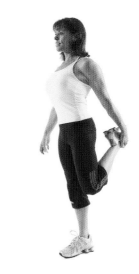

Adductor stretch

- Sit on the floor and place the soles of your feet together.
- Hold on to your ankles and press your thighs down using your elbows.
- Keep your back straight.

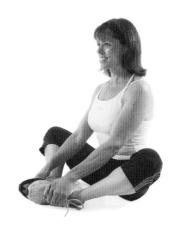

Hamstring stretch

- Sit on the floor with one leg extended and the other leg bent.
- Keeping your back straight and flat, bend forwards from the hips. Reach down towards your foot.
- Flexing your foot will increase the stretch on the calf.
- Repeat on the other side.

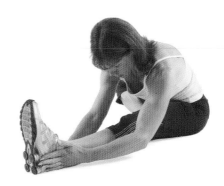

Hip flexor stretch

- From a kneeling position, take a large step forwards so that your knee makes a 90-degree angle and is directly over your foot.
- Keep your body upright and press your rear hip forwards, keeping it square.
- Repeat on the other side.

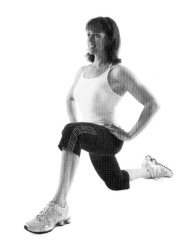

Hips/gluteal/outer thigh stretch

- Sit on the floor with one leg out straight and then cross your other foot over it.
- Place the elbow of the arm on the same side as your straight leg on the outside of the bent knee and slowly look over your shoulder on the side of the bent leg.
- Keep your opposite arm behind your hips for stability.
- Apply pressure to the knee with your elbow.
- Repeat on the other side.

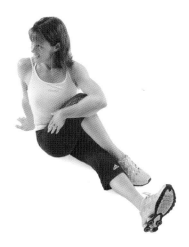

Calf stretch

- From a standing position, take an exaggerated step forwards, keeping your rear leg straight. Hold on to a wall for support if you wish.
- Your front knee should be at 90 degrees and positioned above your foot.
- Lean forwards slightly so that your rear leg and body make a continuous line.
- Repeat on the other side.

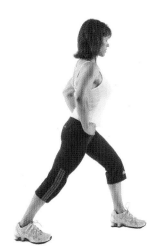

Lower back stretch

- Lie on your back, knees bent and arms straight out to each side.
- Rotate both legs to each side, keeping your head, shoulders and arms in contact with the floor.

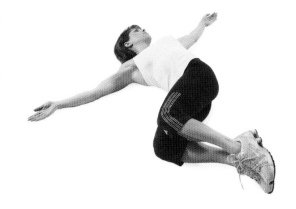

Neck stretch

- Sit erect, head up, then take your hand and gently pull your head towards your shoulder – i.e. so that your ear moves towards your shoulder.
- Apply gentle pressure with your arm over your head.
- Release this pressure before returning your head to the starting position.
- Repeat on the other side.

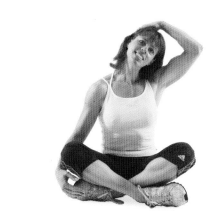

Upper back stretch

- Kneel on the floor.
- Clasp your hands together and push your arms straight out in front of you at shoulder height so you feel a good stretch between the shoulder blades.

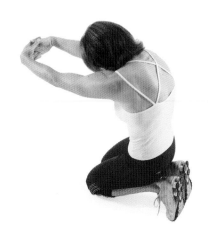

Shoulder stretch

- Grab one elbow with your opposite hand.
- Gently pull it across your body, aiming the elbow towards the opposite shoulder.
- Repeat on the other side.

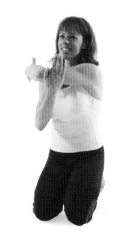

Chest/biceps stretch

- With your arm fully extended, hold on to an upright support at shoulder level. Alternatively, you can use your training partner as support.
- Gently turn your body away from your arm, pressing your shoulder forwards.
- Repeat on the other side.

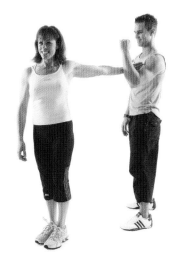

Triceps stretch

- Place one hand between your shoulder blades, hand pointing downwards and elbow pointing upwards.
- Use your opposite hand to gently press down on your right elbow until you feel a stretch in the triceps.
- Repeat on the other side.

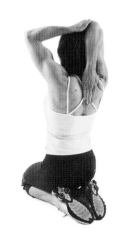

SUMMARY OF KEY POINTS

- Stretching increases flexibility and range of movement, and promotes faster recovery.
- Stretching should be performed only when the muscles are warm.
- Stretching is most beneficial when done between sets and/or after a workout.
- Ease into the stretch, hold and relax, and then gradually release.
- Avoid bouncing and any position of discomfort.
- To improve flexibility, stretches should be held for a minimum of 30 seconds.

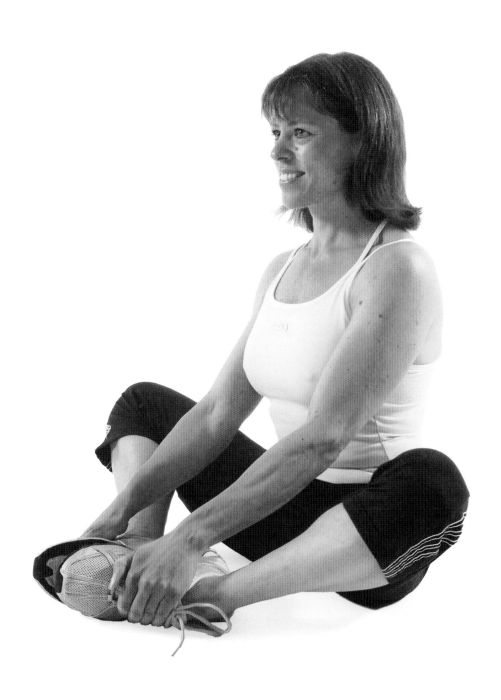

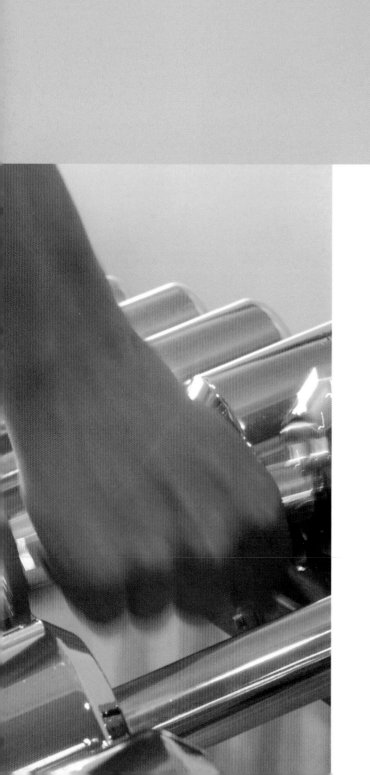

PART **FOUR**

THE WORKOUTS

Finally, here are the workout programmes! There are three basic programmes for beginners, intermediates and advanced trainers, each designed to meet specific fitness and health goals. There are also additional programmes designed to meet different needs, for example to improve performance in different sports or to reduce the risk of injury. All the programmes draw together the scientific theory covered in Parts 1, 2 and 3. Use them as a basis for developing your own individual plan. Happy training!

THE BEGINNER'S PROGRAMME

16

This 12-week programme is designed for those with less than six months of strength training experience or those coming back from a lay-off of longer than three months.

You'll increase your overall fitness and strength, at the same time reducing your body fat levels. The goal of the first three weeks is to introduce your muscles to the stimulus of lifting weights and familiarise you with the exercises.

For the first six weeks, the introductory workout is a circuit routine because you do one set of each exercise with short rests in between. It works all the major muscle groups, and builds a good foundation of strength (or tone) and muscular endurance. The workout contains some of the most effective movements to strengthen muscles for each body part, incorporating compound exercises that work more muscle fibres and through a greater diversity of angles.

From weeks seven to twelve, you'll use what's called a split routine. This is designed to challenge your body more. This phase should lead to noticeable increases in strength, muscle tone and muscular endurance.

You'll no longer be doing a full-body routine; the volume of work is too great to fit into one workout. Instead, you'll split your routine into two workouts and employ the sets training method.

Workout 1 will include upper body exercises for the chest, shoulders and back, while workout 2 will include mostly lower body exercises for the legs as well as for biceps and triceps. Abdominal exercises are included in both workouts.

Q & A

How many reps do I need to do?

During the first 12 weeks, you're aiming to develop muscular endurance rather than size so you should do 12–15 reps per set.

How much weight should I use?

Select weights that allow you to complete the prescribed number of repetitions. The last couple should feel reasonably hard. If 15 reps are easy, you need to use a heavier weight. But don't pile on so much that you're compromising technique. If you cannot complete the set or you feel an intense burn in your muscles, you need to select a lighter weight. To be safe, choose a weight lighter than you think you can do and go from there.

How slowly do I need to go?

Count two seconds up, three seconds down. Lifting weights too fast lets momentum, gravity and other muscles help out, preventing the target muscles from getting the full benefit. The lowering (eccentric) phase of the lift is just as important for building strength and size as the raising (concentric) phase.

How many sets should I do?

For the first six weeks, you do a single set of each exercise before moving on to the next one. Thereafter, in order to continue making gains in strength, you have to step up the workout intensity. Doing three sets of each exercise increases the workload for each body part and is considered effective for maximum development of strength and size.

How long should I rest between workouts?

Rest at least 48 hours before training the same muscle group again. Muscles need time to repair and rebuild themselves. They don't grow during your workout – they rebuild in between workouts, at rest. During the first six weeks when you will be doing a whole-body routine, schedule your workouts every other day – Monday, Wednesday and Friday, for example – to give your muscles time to recuperate. During the sec-

ond six weeks, when you will be doing a split routine, leave at least 48 hours between training the same body part – do workout 1 on Monday and Thursday, and workout 2 on Tuesday and Friday, for example.

BEGINNER'S WORKOUT: WEEKS 1–3

- Complete the following workout twice a week for the first week. If you feel comfortable, increase this to three times a week for the following two weeks.
- Rest for at least one day between workouts.
- Do one circuit for the first week.
- Step up to two circuits in weeks two and three, taking two to three minutes' rest in between.
- Move between exercises with only minimum rest.
- You should complete the workout in well under 30 minutes.

Table 16.1	Beginner's workout: weeks 1–3				
		Week 1		**Weeks 2–3**	
Warm up with a five-minute cardiovascular activity and some mobility movements					
Body part	**Exercise**	**Sets**	**Reps**	**Sets**	**Reps**
Legs	Leg press	1	15	2	15
Chest	Vertical bench press machine	1	15	2	15
Upper back	Machine row	1	15	2	15
Shoulders	Overhead press machine	1	15	2	15
Biceps	Dumbbell curl	1	15	2	15
Triceps	Triceps push-down	1	15	2	15
Lower back	Back extension	1	15	2	15
Abdominals	Crunch	1	15	2	15
Calves	Seated calf raise	1	15	2	15

BEGINNER'S WORKOUT: WEEKS 4–6

- Complete the following workout three times a week.
- Rest for at least one day between workouts.
- Move between exercises with only minimum rest.
- Do two or three circuits with two to three minutes' rest between them.
- You should complete the workout in less than 40 minutes.
- Make sure your technique is sound before increasing the weights.

Concentrate on using a complete range of movement and perfecting your training technique. Don't be tempted to add more sets or push heavy weights. You need to give your body sufficient time to adjust to this type of training. Pushing yourself too hard will not produce greater benefits – recovery times will be lengthened and you may end up overtraining and risking injury.

Table 16.2	Beginner's workout: weeks 4–6		
Body part	**Exercise**	**Sets**	**Reps**
Warm up with a five-minute cardiovascular activity and some mobility movements			
Legs	Leg press	2	15
Hamstrings	Seated leg curl	2	15
Chest	Bench press machine	2	15
Chest	Pec-deck flye	2	15
Upper back	Machine row	2	15
Upper back	Lat pull-down	2	15
Shoulders	Overhead press machine	2	15
Shoulders	Dumbbell lateral raise	2	15
Biceps	Dumbbell curl	2	15
Triceps	Triceps push-down	2	15
Lower back	Back extension	2	15
Abdominals	Crunch	2	15
Calves	Seated calf raise	2	15

BEGINNER'S WORKOUT: WEEKS 7–9

- Complete three workouts per week, alternating workout 1 and workout 2.
- Do three sets of 12 reps of two exercises for chest, upper back and shoulders.
- Do one set of 12 reps for lower back, abdominals, biceps, triceps and calves.
- Rest 30–45 seconds between sets of the same exercise; rest for approximately 60–90 seconds between different exercises.
- Use a heavier weight but maintain strict form.

Table 6.3   Beginner's workout: weeks 7–9 (workout 1)

Body part	Exercise	Sets	Reps
Warm up with a five-minute cardiovascular activity and some mobility movements			
Chest	Dumbbell press	3	12
Chest	Pec-deck flye	3	12
Upper back	Pull-up/chin-up machine	3	12
Upper back	Lat pull-down to front	3	12
Shoulders	Dumbbell press	3	12
Shoulders	Dumbbell lateral raise	3	12
Lower back	Back extension with exercise ball	3	12
Abdominals	Exercise-ball crunch	3	12

Table 6.4   Beginner's workout: weeks 7–9 (workout 2)

Body part	Exercise	Sets	Reps
Warm up with a five-minute cardiovascular activity and some mobility movements			
Legs	Machine squat	3	12
Hamstrings	Seated leg curl	3	12
Quads	Leg extension	3	12
Calves	Standing calf raise	3	12
Biceps	Barbell curl	3	12
Triceps	Bench dip	3	12
Abdominals	Oblique crunch	3	12

BEGINNER'S WORKOUT: WEEKS 10–12

- Complete three workouts per week, alternating workout 1 and workout 2.
- Rest 30–45 seconds between sets of the same exercise; rest for approximately 60–90 seconds between different exercises.

- Do two sets of three exercises for legs, chest and upper back.
- Do two sets of two exercises for shoulders, biceps, triceps, calves and abdominals.

Table 16.5	Beginner's workout: weeks 10–12 (workout 1)		
Body part	**Exercise**	**Sets**	**Reps**
Warm up with a five-minute cardiovascular activity and some mobility movements			
Chest	**Choose three exercises:**	2	12
	Bench press (machine or barbell)		
	Incline dumbbell press		
	Pec-deck flye		
	Dumbbell flye		
Upper back	**Choose three exercises:**	2	12
	Machine row		
	Lat pull-down to front		
	Seated cable row		
	One-arm dumbbell row		
Shoulders	**Choose two exercises:**	2	12
	Overhead press machine		
	Dumbbell lateral raise		
	Dumbbell press		
Lower back	Back extension	3	12
Abdominals	**Choose two exercises:**	2	12
	Crunch (on floor or exercise ball)		
	Oblique crunch		
	Reverse crunch		

Table 16.6	Beginner's workout: weeks 10–12 (workout 2)		
Body part	**Exercise**	**Sets**	**Reps**
Warm up with a five-minute cardiovascular activity and some mobility movements			
Legs	**Choose three exercises:**	2	12
	Leg press machine		
	Machine squat		
	Dumbbell lunge		
	Seated leg curl		
	Leg extension		
	Dumbbell step-ups		
Calves	**Choose two exercises:**	2	12
	Seated calf raise		
	Standing calf raise		
Biceps	**Choose two exercises:**	2	12
	Dumbbell curl		
	Barbell curl		
	Cable curl		
Triceps	**Choose two exercises:**	2	12
	Triceps push-down		
	Bench dips		
	Lying triceps extension		
Abdominals	**Choose two exercises:**	2	12
	Crunch (on floor or exercise ball)		
	Oblique crunch		
	Reverse crunch		

THE INTERMEDIATE'S PROGRAMME

17

This six-month programme is for trainers who have either completed the 12-week beginner's programme or have been training consistently for at least six months.

This programme is designed to increase muscle size and strength, and should be followed for a minimum of six months before progressing to the advanced programme (see pp. 169–75). It includes new exercises to stimulate continued muscle development and a different split routine. The goal is to challenge your body further by working with greater intensity and including more volume.

You'll be training your body over three different workouts instead of two as you did in the final six weeks of the beginner's programme. Workout 1 trains chest and upper back. Workout 2 trains shoulders, biceps and triceps, and workout 3 trains legs, abdominals and lower back. By splitting your body into three parts you can train with even greater intensity and include more volume.

Q & A

How many reps do I need to do?

The number of exercises and sets per body part is increased and you'll now be working in the rep range of eight to twelve. For muscle size and strength, you should do eight to twelve reps per set with 60–90 seconds' rest in between sets. The pyramid training method is used in this programme, so the weight increases and the repetitions decrease progressively with each set (see pp. 135–6).

How much weight should I use?

Choose a weight that will make the last one or two reps challenging. If you can complete 12 reps easily, you need to use a heavier weight. But only increase the weight when you are ready, adding 2.5–5 kg so that you're able to lift only within the eight- to twelve-rep range again.

How slowly do I need to go?

Count two seconds up, three seconds down. Lifting weights too fast lets momentum, gravity and other muscles help out, preventing the target muscles from getting the full benefit. The lowering (eccentric) phase of the lift is just as important for building strength and size as the raising (concentric) phase.

How many sets should I do?

Do three sets of each exercise, although sometimes going under or below this (two to six sets) will produce similar benefits. You'll notice now that as intensity and volume are increased, frequency is gradually decreased. These are important components of a well-designed programme.

How long should I rest between workouts?

Now the volume and intensity has been increased, you'll need more recovery time so you should train each body part only once a week. You could train on Monday, Wednesday and Friday but, if this doesn't suit you, you could choose different days. You have more leeway as to when you train with a three-way training split. While you're doing workout 2, for example, the muscles trained in workout 1 are getting a rest.

Here are two workout programmes, A and B. Follow each for one month (four weeks) then repeat twice so you will have completed the intermediate's programme in six months. The workouts include different exercises, so will keep your body challenged.

INTERMEDIATE'S WORKOUT A

- Complete each workout once a week.
- Rest 60–90 seconds between sets and one to two minutes between exercises.
- Most sets should fall within eight to twelve reps.
- The last repetition of each set should feel extremely hard, and you should be unable to complete another one in proper form.
- Maintain strict form for each repetition, using the complete ROM.

Table 17.1	Intermediate's workout A: workout 1 (chest, upper back, abdominals)		
Body part	**Exercise**	**Sets**	**Reps**
Warm up with a five-minute cardiovascular activity and some mobility movements			
Chest	Bench press (barbell)	3	8–12
	Incline dumbbell press	3	8–12
	Cable cross-over	2	8–12
Upper back	One-arm dumbbell row	3	8–12
	Lat pull-down to front	3	8–12
	Seated cable row	2	8–12
Abdominals	Reverse crunch*	3	12–15
	Crunch*	3	12–15

* Perform as a superset – do the first exercise immediately followed by the second exercise. Rest for one to two minutes before repeating the superset.

Table 17.2	Intermediate's workout A: workout 2 (shoulders, arms, abdominals)		
Body part	**Exercise**	**Sets**	**Reps**
Warm up with a five-minute cardiovascular activity and some mobility movements			
Shoulders	Dumbbell press	3	8–12
	Dumbbell lateral raise	3	8–12
	Bent-over lateral raise	2	8–12
Biceps	Barbell curl	2	8–12
	Concentration curl	2	8–12
Triceps	Triceps push-down	2	8–12
	Lying triceps extension	2	8–12
Abdominals	Oblique crunch*	3	12–15
	Plank*	3	Hold for 60–120 seconds

* Perform as a superset – do the first exercise immediately followed by the second exercise. Rest for one to two minutes before repeating the superset.

Table 17.3	Intermediate's workout A: workout 3 (legs, abdominals, lower back)		
Body part	**Exercise**	**Sets**	**Reps**
Warm up with a five-minute cardiovascular activity and some mobility movements			
Legs	Split squat	3	8–12
	Dead lift	3	8–12
	Leg extension	2	8–12
	Seated leg curl	2	8–12
Calves	Seated calf raise	3	12–15
Abdominals	Exercise ball pull-in*	3	12–15
	Side bridge*	3	5**
Lower back	Back extension with exercise ball	3	12–15

* Perform as a superset – do the first exercise immediately followed by the second exercise. Rest for one to two minutes before repeating the superset.

** Hold for five seconds, repeat for five reps on each side.

INTERMEDIATE'S WORKOUT B

- Complete each workout once a week.
- Rest 60–90 seconds between sets and one to two minutes between exercises.
- Most sets should fall within eight to twelve reps.
- The last repetition of each set should feel extremely hard, and you should be unable to complete another one in proper form.
- Maintain strict form for each repetition, using the complete ROM.

Table 17.4	Intermediate's workout B: workout I (chest, upper back, abdominals)		
Body part	**Exercise**	**Sets**	**Reps**
Warm up with a five-minute cardiovascular activity and some mobility movements			
Chest	Dumbbell press	3	8–12
	Incline dumbbell flye	3	8–12
	Exercise ball press-up	2	8–12
Upper back	Pull-up ('chins')	3	8–12
	Dumbbell pull-over	3	8–12
	Dumbbell shrug	2	8–12
Abdominals	Exercise ball crunch*	3	12–15
	Side crunch*	3	12–15

* Perform as a superset – do the first exercise immediately followed by the second exercise. Rest for one to two minutes before repeating the superset.

Table 17.5	Intermediate's workout B: workout 2 (shoulders, arms, abdominals)		
Body part	**Exercise**	**Sets**	**Reps**
Warm up with a five-minute cardiovascular activity and some mobility movements			
Shoulders	Overhead press machine	3	8–12
	Upright row	3	8–12
	Bent-over lateral raise	2	8–12
Biceps	EZ-bar curl	2	8–12
	Incline dumbbell curl	2	8–12
Triceps	Bench dip	2	8–12
	Triceps kickback	2	8–12
Abdominals	Crunch*	3	12–15
	Alternate twisting exercise ball crunch*	3	12–15

* Perform as a superset – do the first exercise immediately followed by the second exercise. Rest for one to two minutes before repeating the superset.

Table 17.6	Intermediate's workout B: workout 3 (legs, abdominals, lower back)		
Body part	**Exercise**	**Sets**	**Reps**
Warm up with a five-minute cardiovascular activity and some mobility movements			
Legs	Leg press	3	8–12
	Machine squats	3	8–12
	Front lunge	2	8–12
	Reverse lunge	2	8–12
Calves	Standing calf raise (Smith machine)	3	12–15
Abdominals	Reverse crunch*	3	12–15
	Hip thrust*	3	12–15
Lower back	Back extension with rotation	3	12–15

* Perform as a superset – do the first exercise immediately followed by the second exercise. Rest for one to two minutes before repeating the superset.

THE ADVANCED PROGRAMME

18

This advanced programme is a progression of the intermediate's programme. It provides a more serious workout for trainers who have completed the intermediate's programme, have trained consistently for at least a year, and are looking to add a greater variety of exercises and training techniques to their workouts.

The goal is to further overload your muscles to increase muscle strength and size. Thus it provides a higher-intensity workout. This programme is based on a similar three-way split workout to the intermediate workout but incorporates advanced training techniques – descending sets, supersets and pre-exhaustion – alongside the established basic methods of sets and pyramid training.

You can include an advanced technique once a week or once every two weeks. However, as they are very intense, you should avoid using these techniques too frequently on any one body part as they impose considerable stress on the muscles.

Q & A

How often should I do an advanced workout?

Choose one of following advanced workouts in place of your regular (intermediate) workout (see the periodisation chart on p. 182) once every two weeks. Do not use an advanced training technique on the same body part more frequently than once a fortnight otherwise you risk overtraining.

How much weight should I use?

Choose a weight that will make the last one or two reps challenging. If you can complete 12 reps easily, you need to use a heavier weight. Only increase the weight when you are ready, adding 2.5–5 kg so that you're able to lift only within the eight- to twelve-rep range again.

How slowly do I need to go?

Count two seconds up, three seconds down. Lifting weights too fast lets momentum, gravity and other muscles help out, preventing the target muscles from getting the full benefit. The lowering (eccentric) phase of the lift is just as important for building strength and size as the raising (concentric) phase.

How many sets should I do?

You should do approximately eight sets for legs, upper back, chest and shoulders, and four sets for biceps, triceps, calves and lower back.

How long should I rest between workouts?

Each body part should be trained just once a week to allow sufficient recovery time between workouts. Ideally, you should train on non-consecutive days, but with a three-way training split, you have some leeway – the muscles trained in the previous workout are getting a rest while you perform your next workout.

DESCENDING SETS

Complete the first two sets of the exercise, performing eight to twelve reps per set, then do a descending set for your last set. Complete eight to twelve reps in good form, then reduce the weight by 20–30 per cent and immediately complete as many repetitions as possible until you reach 'failure'. You should be able to complete an additional four to eight reps. If you wish, you can reduce the weight a further 20–30 per cent and complete as many reps as you can. Take two to three minutes' rest between sets and between exercises.

Table 18.1	Advanced workout 1 with descending sets (chest, arms)		
Body part	**Exercise**	**Sets**	**Reps**
Warm up with a five-minute cardiovascular activity and some mobility movements			
Chest	Bench press (barbell or dumbbell)	3	8–12
	Incline bench press (barbell or dumbbell)	3	8–12 3rd set descending set
	Dumbbell flye (flat or incline)	2	8–12 2nd set descending set
Biceps	Dumbbell curl	2	8–12 3rd set descending set
	Concentration curl	2	8–12
Triceps	Lying triceps extension	2	8–12 2nd set descending set
	Reverse-grip triceps press-down	2	8–12
Abdominals	Oblique crunch*	2	12–15
	Hanging leg raise*	2	12–15

* Perform as a superset – do the first exercise immediately followed by the second exercise. Rest for one to two minutes before repeating the superset.

Table 18.2	Advanced workout 2 with descending sets (shoulders, back)		
Body part	**Exercise**	**Sets**	**Reps**
Warm up with a five-minute cardiovascular activity and some mobility movements			
Shoulders	Dumbbell press	3	8–12
	Dumbbell lateral raise	3	8–12
			3rd set descending set
	Upright row	2	8–12
			2nd set descending set
Upper back	Barbell row	3	8–12
			3rd set descending set
	Pull-up/chin-up	3	8–12
			3rd set descending set
	Straight-arm pull-down	2	8–12
Abdominals	Exercise ball crunch*	2	12–15
	Hip thrust*	2	12–15

* Perform as a superset – do the first exercise immediately followed by the second exercise. Rest for one to two minutes before repeating the superset.

Table 18.3	Advanced workout 3 with descending sets (legs)		
Body part	**Exercise**	**Sets**	**Reps**
Warm up with a five-minute cardiovascular activity and some mobility movements			
Quadriceps/gluteals	Squat	3	8–12
Quadriceps	Leg extension	3	8–12
			3rd set descending set
Hamstrings	Straight-leg dead lift	3	8–12
			3rd set descending set
Calves	Seated calf raise	3	8–12
			3rd set descending set
Abdominals	Exercise ball pull-in*	2	12–15
	Side bridge*	2	5**

* Perform as a superset – do the first exercise immediately followed by the second exercise. Rest for one to two minutes before repeating the superset.

** Hold for five seconds, repeat five times on each side.

SUPERSETS

Pair exercises are mirror images of each other, like leg extensions and leg curls. Do the first exercise of the superset first (e.g. barbell bent-over row), followed immediately by the second exercise (e.g. bench press). That is one superset. Rest for one to two minutes then repeat the process. Once you complete the prescribed number of supersets, rest for two minutes then move on to the next superset.

Table 18.4	Advanced workout 2 with supersets (chest, back, shoulders)		
Body part	**Exercise**	**Sets**	**Reps**
Warm up with a five-minute cardiovascular activity and some mobility movements			
Chest and back			
Superset No. 1			
Back	Barbell bent-over row	3	8–12
Chest	Bench press		8–12
Superset No. 2			
Back	Lat pull-down	3	8–12
Chest	Incline dumbbell press		8–12
Shoulders and trapezius			
Superset No. 3			
Shoulders	Dumbbell press	3	8–12
Trapezius	Upright row		8–12
Superset No. 4			
Shoulders	Lateral raise	3	8–12
Trapezius	Dumbbell shrug		8–12

Table 18.5	Advanced workout 2 with supersets (quadriceps/hamstrings and calves/forearms)		
Body part	**Exercise**	**Sets**	**Reps**
Warm up with a five-minute cardiovascular activity and some mobility movements			
Quadriceps and hamstrings			
Superset No. 1			
Quadriceps	Squat	3	8–12
Hamstrings	Straight-leg dead lift		8–12
Superset No. 2			
Quadriceps	Leg extension	3	8–12
Hamstrings	Seated leg curl		8–12
Calves and forearms			
Superset No. 3			
Calves	Standing calf raise	3	8–12
Forearms	Wrist curl		8–12

Table 18.6	Advanced workout 3 with supersets (biceps/triceps and abdominals/lower back)		
Body part	**Exercise**	**Sets**	**Reps**
Warm up with a five-minute cardiovascular activity and some mobility movements			
Biceps and triceps			
Superset No. 1			
Biceps	Barbell curl	3	8–12
Triceps	Triceps push-down		8–12
Superset No. 2			
Biceps	Preacher curl	3	8–12
Triceps	Bench dip		8–12
Abdominals and lower back			
Superset No. 3			
Abdominals	Crunch	3	15–20
Lower back	Back extension with exercise ball		15–20
Abdominals and lower back			
Superset No. 4			
Abdominals	Reverse crunch	3	15–20
Lower back	Back extension with rotation		15–20

PRE-EXHAUSTION

The pre-exhaustion training method is used for chest, shoulders and legs. An isolation exercise is performed followed by a compound exercise. Rest 60–90 seconds between sets and two to three minutes between exercises.

Table 18.7	Advanced workout 1 with pre-exhaustion (chest, back, shoulders)		
Body part	Exercise	Sets	Reps
Warm up with a five-minute cardiovascular activity and some mobility movements			
Chest	Dumbbell flye	4	8–12
	Bench press (barbell or dumbbell)	4	8–12
Shoulders	Dumbbell lateral raise	4	8–12
	Dumbbell press/overhead press machine	4	8–12
Abdominals	Exercise ball pull-in*	3	12–15
	Side bridge*	3	5**

* Perform as a superset – do the first exercise immediately followed by the second exercise. Rest for one to two minutes before repeating the superset.

** Hold for five seconds, repeat for five reps on each side.

Table 18.8	Day 2: advanced workout 2 with pre-exhaustion (legs)		
Body part	Exercise	Sets	Reps
Warm up with a five-minute cardiovascular activity and some mobility movements			
Quadriceps	Leg extension	3	8–12
Hamstrings	Lying leg curl	3	8–12
Quadriceps/hamstrings, gluteals	Leg press	4	8–12
Calves	Standing calf raise	3	8–12
Abdominals	Exercise ball crunch*	3	12–15
	Alternate twisting exercise ball crunch*	3	12–15

* Perform as a superset – do the first exercise immediately followed by the second exercise. Rest for one to two minutes before repeating the superset.

Table 18.9	Day 3: advanced workout 3 with pre-exhaustion (upper back, biceps, triceps)		
Body part	**Exercise**	**Sets**	**Reps**
Warm up with a five-minute cardiovascular activity and some mobility movements			
Upper back	Lat pull-down	3	8–12
	Seated row	3	8–12
	Dumbbell shrug	2	8–12
Biceps	Barbell curl	2	8–12
	Concentration curl	2	8–12
Triceps	Lying triceps extension	2	8–12
	Triceps push-down	2	8–12
Abdominals	Oblique crunch*	3	12–15
	Plank*	3	Hold for 60–120 seconds
Lower back	Back extension with rotation	3	12–15

* Perform as a superset – do the first exercise immediately followed by the second exercise. Rest for one to two minutes before repeating the superset.

THE STRENGTH PROGRAMME

19

The aim of this programme is to increase pure strength. In addition to power lifters, anyone training for muscle size would benefit from including a maximum-strength phase in their training cycle (see the section on periodisation, pp. 180–84). It can help you get through a sticking point by allowing you to lift more weight and further increase your muscle size when you resume your regular routine. The idea is that by varying the intensity, you alter the recruitment of muscle fibres so that, over time, you recruit more fibres.

Training for strength involves using basic compound exercises – squats, dead lifts and bench presses – with heavy weights and low reps. This type of training causes maximum stimulation of the powerful FT muscle fibres and hence greater muscle strength. It not only increases muscle strength but also improves joint stability and muscle mass.

Q & A

How long can I follow this workout?

You can incorporate this strength programme into your bodybuilding programme for a period of four to six weeks, in place of your normal workouts. After this, return to your normal routine.

How often should I train?

Do the workout twice a week.

How much weight should I use?

Using near-maximal weights – at least 85 per cent 1RM – develops maximum strength. If you do not know your 1RM, find a weight that you can just lift for six strict repetitions. This will approximate to 70–80 per cent 1RM. As with any bodybuilding programme, you need to increase the weight you lift gradually over time.

Any precautions?

It is important to warm up thoroughly otherwise you risk injury. Perform five minutes of a cardiovascular activity followed by two or three sets of that exercise using very light weights for about 15 reps before embarking on the heavy sets. Ensure that you use the full ROM for each exercise and train using perfect technique.

How many sets and reps?

Following your warm-up sets, perform four working sets of each exercise. Begin with weights equal to 70–80 per cent of your 1RM and do six to eight reps. Progress to 80–90 per cent of your 1RM for three to four reps. You should also allow longer rest periods between sets (three to four minutes) than in the bodybuilding programme to allow full recovery of your fuel system.

Table 19.1	Strength workout 1 (legs, back)		
Body part	**Exercise**	**Sets**	**Reps**
Warm up with a five-minute cardiovascular activity and some mobility movements			
Legs	Squat	4	8, 6, 3–4, 3–4
	Dead lift	4	8, 6, 3–4, 3–4
Upper back	Bent-over row	4	8, 6, 3–4, 3–4
	Lat pull-down	4	8, 6, 3–4, 3–4
Abdominals	Crunch	2	12–15
	Hanging leg raise	2	12–15

Table 19.2	Strength workout 2 (chest, shoulders, arms)		
Body part	**Exercise**	**Sets**	**Reps**
Warm up with a five-minute cardiovascular activity and some mobility movements			
Chest	Bench press	4	8, 6, 3–4, 3–4
	Incline dumbbell press	4	8, 6, 3–4, 3–4
Shoulders	Dumbbell press	4	8, 6, 3–4, 3–4
	Upright row	4	8, 6, 3–4, 3–4
Abdominals	Oblique crunch	2	12–15
	Exercise ball jack-knife	2	12–15

THE PERIODISATION PROGRAMME

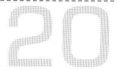

Periodisation refers to the planned manipulation of training volume and intensity throughout a series of specific training phases or cycles. It is an application of the principles of progressive training (you vary your repetitions, sets, weight and intensity during each cycle) and is a method used to make continual improvements in performance throughout the year, thus avoiding reaching plateaux. If you follow the same workout for any length of time, the body soon adapts to the constant load and your gains diminish. However, by structuring your long-term training goals in a number of training cycles, you will be able to make gains in strength, mass and definition all year round, and will also avoid overtraining and injury.

Proof that periodisation works better than sticking to the same routine week after week comes from a study at Appalachian State University in Boone, North Carolina, and the USA Weightlifting Development Center in Shreveport, Louisiana.[1] The experienced weight trainers who followed a periodised programme made significant improvements in strength (as measured by their 1RM for the squat), whereas those who followed a standard programme did not show any improvement.

A periodisation programme is divided into a number of distinct cycles.[2] The longest cycle is called a macrocycle and usually spans a period of one year, although shorter macrocycles can be used – for example, two macrocycles per year are used in a double-periodisation programme. This would suit those who cannot commit themselves to a year-round programme or those who want greater variety in their training.

The year is then broken down into two to six shorter training cycles (mesocycles), each spanning several weeks. Each mesocycle emphasises a particular training goal (e.g. muscle size or muscular endurance) and involves a gradual increase in training intensity. The aim is to peak at the end of your mesocycle. For strength trainers, this may be gauged by the amount of weight that can be lifted.

Each mesocycle is then followed by a short period (one to two weeks) of relative rest, which is important to allow your body to recover and recuperate before beginning the next mesocycle. Provided this rest phase lasts no longer than four weeks, you will not experience a detraining effect (see also p. 144). During this time, you should do only very light training, or a completely different activity such as golf or recreational swimming that does not tax your energy systems or central nervous system in the same way.

Each mesocycle is then divided into week-long microcycles, around which you plan your day-to-day workouts.

There are many variations on periodisation programmes, dependent on your goals, training experience and lifestyle. The examples given on the following pages may be used as a basis for designing your own programme. You may commence training at any time during the year – simply change the month headings. The important point is to follow the mesocycles in the given order, and to gradually increase your training intensity within each mesocycle.

PERIODISATION PROGRAMME 1: MUSCULAR ENDURANCE

Aims

1. Improve muscular endurance
2. Improve muscle tone

This periodisation programme emphasises muscular endurance and comprises four mesocycles of circuit training, each progressively increasing in intensity. Shortening the rest intervals from 30 seconds to 20 seconds, adding more circuits to your allocated workout time, and changing the reps and weight achieve this. If you are training for a particular sport, include exercises that work the main muscle groups involved in that sport and that also mimic the movements used (e.g. lat pull-down if you are a swimmer). You can also concentrate on particular goals:

- muscular strength and endurance – use slightly heavier weights for 12–15 reps, with slightly longer rest intervals between exercises
- cardiovascular fitness/fat loss – use lighter weights for up to 20 reps, with a cardiovascular exercise such as the stationary bike or jogging between stations.

Table 20.1 Periodisation programme 1 – to improve muscular endurance (beginners)

						Macrocycle						
Jan.	Feb.	Mar.	Apr.	May	June	July	Aug.	Sept.	Oct.	Nov.	Dec.	
Mesocycle 1			Mesocycle 2			Mesocycle 3			Mesocycle 4			
12 weeks ME		1 week R	12 weeks ME		1 week R	12 weeks ME		1 week R	12 weeks ME		1 week R	

Progression

- Reduce rest interval between sets from 30 to 15 seconds
- Increase repetitions from 15 to a maximum of 20
- Increase number of circuits performed in 45 minutes
- Use slightly heavier weights if you can exceed 20 reps

Key:
ME = muscle endurance training (see p. 143)
R = rest/low-intensity activity

PERIODISATION PROGRAMME 2: MUSCLE SIZE (BEGINNERS)

Aims

1. Increase muscle size
2. Increase strength

This cycle includes a 12-week muscular endurance meso-cycle to build a good base of conditioning and prepare the muscles for the next mesocycles. The exact length of the muscle size mesocycles will depend on your level of conditioning and any holiday commitments. For example, you may need to shorten mesocycle 1 to avoid overtraining. As you become progressively adapted to training, however, you should be able to sustain the full training cycles. Increase the intensity gradually by using progressively heavier weights.

Table 20.2 Periodisation programme 2 – to improve muscle size (beginners)

Jan.	Feb.	Mar.	Apr.	May	June	July	Aug.	Sept.	Oct.	Nov.	Dec.
Mesocycle 1			Mesocycle 2			Mesocycle 3			Mesocycle 4		
12 weeks ME		1 week R	10 weeks ME		3 week R	10 weeks ME		3 week R	4 weeks MS	2 weeks AMS	4 weeks MS
									2 weeks AMS		1 week R

Macrocycle

Progression

- Gradually increase weight used in each mesocycle

Key:
ME = muscle endurance training (see p. 143)
MS = muscle size training (see pp. 165–6)
AMS = advanced muscle size training (see pp. 170–5 – descending (drop) set workout)
R = rest/low-intensity activity

PERIODISATION PROGRAMME 3: MUSCLE SIZE (INTERMEDIATE AND ADVANCED)

Aims

1. Increase muscle size
2. Increase strength

This plan is suitable for weight trainers with at least one to two years' training experience. Following a six-week meso-cycle building muscle endurance and strength, this periodisation programme emphasises muscle hypertrophy. Muscle size cycles dominate, interspersed with short periods that incorporate advanced training methods – descending (drop) sets, supersets and pre-exhaustion – and maximum strength training methods. The objective of this approach is to avoid training plateaux and produce long-term muscle size gains.

Table 20.3 Periodisation programme 3 – to improve muscle size (advanced)

	Jan.	Feb.	Mar.	Apr.	May	June	July	Aug.	Sept.	Oct.	Nov.	Dec.
Macrocycle												
	Mesocycle 1			Mesocycle 2			Mesocycle 3			Mesocycle 4		
Weeks	6 weeks	1 week R	6 weeks	1 week R	6 weeks	2 wks	4 weeks	1 week R / 2 wks	4 weeks	4 weeks	4 weeks	4 weeks / 1 week R
Type	ME	R	MS	R	MS	AMS	MS	R / AMS	MS	MS	MS	MXS / R

Progression

- Gradually increase amount of weight used

Key:
ME = muscle endurance training (see pp. 167–8)
MS = muscle size training (see p. 165–6)
AMS = advanced muscle size training (see pp. 170–5 – any of the three workouts)
MXS = maximum strength training (see pp. 176–7)
R = rest/low-intensity activity

PERIODISATION PROGRAMME 4: MAXIMUM STRENGTH (ADVANCED)

Aims

1. Increase maximum strength
2. Promote long-term hypertrophy

This periodisation programme is suitable for advanced weight trainers who want to develop stronger muscles and long-term hypertrophy. Following a six-week conditioning mesocycle to prepare the body for the forthcoming intense training, it incorporates both maximum strength training methods as well as advanced muscle size training methods. Muscle strength training cycles dominate and are interspersed with advanced training method cycles and maximum strength training.

Table 20.4 Periodisation programme 4 – to increase maximum strength (advanced)

						Macrocycle						
Jan.	Feb.	Mar.	Apr.	May	June	July	Aug.	Sept.	Oct.	Nov.	Dec.	
Mesocycle 1		Mesocycle 2		Mesocycle 3			Mesocycle 4			Mesocycle 5		
6 weeks	1 week R	6 weeks	6 weeks	1 week R	6 weeks	3 weeks	2 week R	3 weeks	3weeks	3 weeks	1 week R	4 weeks	2wks	3 weeks	2 week R
ME		MS	MXS		MXS	AMS		MS	MXS	AMS		MXS	AMS	MXS	

Progression

- Gradually increase amount of weight used

Key:
ME = muscle endurance training (see pp. 167–8)
MS = muscle size training (see pp. 165–6)
AMS = advanced muscle size training (see pp. 170–5 – any of the three workouts)
MXS = maximum strength training (see pp. 176–7)
R = rest/low-intensity activity

TRAINING FOR SPORTS PROGRAMMES

21

While fitness athletes and bodybuilders train primarily to change the appearance of their physiques, other athletes can tailor a strength training programme to improve various aspects of their sports performance.

Weight training can help to:
- improve sports performance
- improve strength, power, muscle size or muscular endurance
- reduce injury risk.

When designing a sports strength training programme, however, it has to be specific to the requirements of your sport. You need to consider the following:
- the movement patterns of your sport, and which muscles are used
- the relative importance of strength, power, hypertrophy and muscular endurance in your sport
- which muscles or joints are most prone to injury and therefore need strengthening
- the priorities of your sport's season – i.e. off-season, pre-season, in-season and post-season
- Your fitness level and training experience.

THE ATHLETE'S (SPRINTER'S) WORKOUT

Goal

This workout includes exercises for each muscle group, with a particular emphasis on compound

---

General guidelines for strength training for sport

1. Use different programmes for each season, focusing on developing only one of these goals (e.g. strength). Attempting to improve in two or more areas (e.g. strength and muscular endurance) simultaneously will produce only mediocre improvements.

2. During the off-season focus on developing your strength and hypertrophy.

3. Pre-season training should focus on one particular fitness aspect (e.g. power, muscular endurance or strength) that is relevant to the sport. Use one of the programmes detailed in the first part of this chapter.

4. During the season, concentrate on maintaining your fitness and staying injury-free. The frequency and duration of your strength training workouts should be reduced and the exercises should be more sport-specific.

5. Include mostly compound exercises in your programme. They will improve your balance and coordination while increasing strength. Keep isolation exercises to a minimum and schedule these at the end of your workout.

6. Keep rest periods fairly short (between 60 and 90 seconds) to mimic the demands of your sport.

7. Choose a weight with which the set becomes difficult by the last one or two repetitions.

8. Maintain strict form for each repetition, using the complete ROM.

9. Emphasise quality rather than quantity.

Table 21.1	Priorities for a sport-specific strength training programme		
Season	**Sports-specific training**	**Strength training**	**Strength-training goal**
Off-season	Low	High	Hypertrophy and strength
Pre-season	Medium	Medium	Strength/power/ muscular endurance – depending on the sport
In-season	High	Low	Maintain strength/ power/muscular endurance

Table 21.2	Athlete's (sprinter's) workout		
Muscle group	**Exercise**	**Sets**	**Reps**
Workout 1 (lower body)			
Quadriceps/gluteals	Squat	2–3	8–12
	Dead lift	2–3	8–12
Quadriceps/gluteals/ hamstrings	Lunge (front or reverse)	2	8–12
Hamstrings	Straight-leg dead lift	2	8–12
Calves	Standing calf raise	3	8–12
Abdominals	Crunch	2	15–20
	Hanging leg raise	2	15–20
Workout 2 (upper body)			
Chest	Bench press (flat or incline)	2–3	8–12
Back	Bent-over row	2–3	8–12
Shoulders	Shoulder press (barbell/dumbbell)	2–3	8–12
Biceps	Barbell curl	2	8–12
Triceps	Lying triceps extension	2	8–12
Trapezius	Dumbbell shrug	2	8–12
Lower back	Back extension	2	12–15
Abdominals	Alternate twisting exercise ball crunch	2	15–20
	Plank	2	Hold for 60 s

exercises, to cause maximum muscle stimulation. There is equal emphasis on lower- and upper-body exercises to build balanced muscle development. Moderate to heavy weights should be used, and the prescribed sets and reps are designed to develop muscle strength and hypertrophy.

How many reps?

Eight to twelve reps per set with 60–90 seconds' rest in between sets.

How much weight?

Choose a weight that will make the last one or two reps challenging.

How slowly?

Count two seconds up, three seconds down.

How many sets?

Do two or three sets of each exercise.

How much rest between workouts?

Weight train three times a week with at least a day's rest in between, alternating workout 1 (lower body) and workout 2 (upper body).

In-season guidelines

As the competitive season approaches, reduce the number of weight training sessions to twice a week and increase the time spent on sport-specific training.

Increase the number of repetitions to 12–15 to emphasise muscle endurance.

Include plyometrics and jump exercises after a good warm-up then follow with strength exercises. Do approximately 10 reps per set with a three- to five-minute rest between sets.

THE FOOTBALLER'S WORKOUT

Goal

This workout aims to develop overall strength and hypertrophy. It therefore includes exercises for each muscle group to promote balanced development, as all muscles are important in football. Rather more emphasis (in the form of more sets) is placed on exercises for the lower body, in particular exercises for the hamstrings, than the upper body.

How many reps?

Eight to twelve reps per set with 60–90 seconds' rest in between sets.

How much weight?

Choose a moderate-heavy weight that will make the last one or two reps challenging.

How slowly?

Count two seconds up, three seconds down.

How many sets?

Do three sets of each exercise.

How much rest between workouts?

Weight train three times a week with at least a day's rest in between, alternating workout 1 (lower body) and workout 2 (upper body).

Table 21.3	Footballer's workout		
Muscle group	**Exercise**	**Sets**	**Reps**
Workout 1 (lower body)			
Quadriceps/gluteals	Leg press	3	8–12
Quadriceps	Leg extension	3	8–12
Hamstrings	Seated leg curl	3	8–12
Calves	Standing calf raise	3	8–12
Lower back	Back extension	2	12–15
Abdominals	Exercise ball crunch	2	15–20
	Hanging leg raise	2	15–20
Workout 2 (upper body)			
Chest	Bench press (flat or incline)	3	8–12
Back	Lat pull-down	3	8–12
Shoulders	Dumbbell shoulder press	3	8–12
Triceps	Lying triceps extension	3	8–12
Biceps	Barbell curl	3	8–12
Abdominals	Oblique crunch	2	12–15
	Exercise ball jack-knife	2	12–15

In-season guidelines

As the competitive season approaches, reduce the number of weight training sessions to twice a week and increase the time spent on sport-specific training.

Reduce the number of sets per body part and increase the number of repetitions to 12–15 to emphasise muscle endurance.

Include plyometrics and jump exercises after a good warm-up then follow with strength exercises. Do approximately 10 reps per set with a three- to five-minute rest between sets.

THE SWIMMER'S WORKOUT

Goal

This workout aims to develop muscular and cardiovascular endurance as well as some strength.

It emphasises exercises for the upper body, since arm action is the most important action for generating speed in swimming, and exercises for the mid-section as these muscles are important for maintaining the straight-body water position. It also includes a plyometric exercise for legs to help improve the explosive power needed for push-offs.

How many reps?

For general conditioning, do 12–15 reps per set with 30–60 seconds' rest in between sets. Sprinters may wish to do fewer reps and use heavier weights to build strength; long-distance swimmers may wish to do a higher number of reps, around 15–20.

Table 21.4	Swimmer's workout		
Muscle group	Exercise	Sets	Reps
Back	Straight-arm pull-down	3	12–15
	Dumbbell pull-over	3	12–15
Shoulders	Bent-over lateral raise	3	12–15
	Dumbbell lateral raise	3	12–15
Biceps	Barbell curl	2	12–15
Triceps	Triceps press-down	2	12–15
Lower back	Back extension	2	12–15
Lower body	Squat jumps (with or without dumbbells)	2	10–12
Abdominals	Reverse crunch	2	15–20
	Alternate twisting exercise ball crunch	2	15–20
	Exercise ball pull-in	2	15–20

How much weight?

Choose a moderate weight that will make the last one or two reps challenging.

How slowly?

Count two seconds up, three seconds down.

How many sets?

Do three sets of each exercise.

How much rest between workouts?

Weight train three times a week with at least a day's rest in between.

In-season guidelines

As the competitive season approaches, reduce the number of weight training sessions to twice a week and increase the time spent on sport-specific training – movements that duplicate the movement patterns of each stroke – and in the pool.

You can adapt many weight training exercises to mimic the actions in a particular stroke more closely.

Include more plyometric exercises after a good warm-up then follow with strength exercises. Do approximately 10 reps per set with a three- to five-minute rest between sets.

THE RUGBY PLAYER'S WORKOUT

Goal

Rugby players require considerable strength, power and speed as well as endurance. This workout focuses on strength, power and hypertrophy, and includes basic compound exercises for both upper and lower body to promote balanced development.

Table 21.5	Rugby player's workout		
Muscle group	**Exercise**	**Sets**	**Reps**
Workout 1 (lower body, back)			
Lower body	Squat	3	6–10
	Dead lift	3	6–10
Quadriceps	Leg extension	2	6–10
Hamstrings	Lying leg curl	2	6–10
Calves	Standing calf raise	3	6–10
	Seated calf raise	3	6–10
Back	Bent-over barbell row	3	
	Pull-up/chin-up	3	6–10
Lower back	Back extension	2	12–15
Abdominals	Exercise ball crunch	2	12–15
	Reverse crunch	2	12–15
Workout 2 (chest, shoulders, arms)			
Chest	Bench press	3	6–10
	Incline dumbbell press	3	6–10
Shoulders	Dumbbell shoulder press	3	6–10
	Upright row	3	6–10
Triceps	Lying triceps extension	3	6–10
Biceps	Barbell curl	3	6–10
Abdominals	Oblique crunch	2	12–15
	Exercise ball pull-in	2	12–15

How many reps?

Six to ten reps per set with 60–90 seconds' rest in between sets.

How much weight?

Select a heavy weight that will make the last one or two reps challenging.

How slowly?

Count two seconds up, three seconds down.

How many sets?

Do two or three sets of each exercise.

How much rest between workouts?

Weight train three times a week with at least a day's rest in between, alternating workout 1 (lower body) and workout 2 (upper body).

Table 21.6	Runner's workout		
Muscle group	Exercise	Sets	Reps
Legs	Split squat	2	12–15
	Step-ups	2	12–15
Calves	Calf raise	2	12–15
Chest	Dumbbell flye	2	12–15
Shoulders	Dumbbell lateral raise	2	12–15
Back	Lat pull-down	2	12–15
Biceps	Dumbbell curl	2	12–15
Triceps	Triceps press-down	2	12–15
Lower back	Back extension	2	12–15
Abdominals	Reverse crunch	2	15–20
	Plank	2	Hold for 60–90 s

In-season guidelines

As the competitive season approaches, reduce the number of weight training sessions to twice a week and increase the time spent on sport-specific training.

Reduce the number of sets per body part and increase the number of repetitions to 12–15 to emphasise muscle endurance.

Include plyometric and jump exercises after a good warm-up then follow with strength exercises. Do approximately 10 reps per set with a three- to five-minute rest between sets.

THE RUNNER'S WORKOUT

Goal

The aim of this workout is to improve overall conditioning. It develops your muscular and cardiovascular endurance and provides a balanced workout to help avoid the overuse injuries that are common in running.

How many reps?

Do 12–15 reps per set with 30–60 seconds' rest in between sets.

How much weight?

Choose a light-moderate weight that will make the last one or two reps challenging.

How slowly?

Count two seconds up, three seconds down.

How many sets?

Do two sets of each exercise.

How much rest between workouts?

Weight train two or three times a week with at least a day's rest in between.

Table 21.7	Cyclist's workout		
Muscle group	**Exercise**	**Sets**	**Reps**
Shoulders	Overhead press machine	3	12–15
Back	Lat pull-down	3	12–15
Chest	Vertical bench press machine	3	12–15
Legs	Front or reverse lunge	3	12–15
Hamstrings	Seated leg curl	3	12–15
Lower back	Back extension	2	12–15
Calves	Seated calf raise	3	12–15
Abdominals	Exercise ball crunch	2	15–20
	Hip thrust	2	15–20

In-season guidelines

As the competitive season approaches, reduce the number of weight training sessions to twice a week and increase running training.

Increase the number of reps and reduce the weights.

THE CYCLIST'S WORKOUT

Goal

The aim of this workout is to increase your muscular and cardiovascular endurance. It includes exercises for both the upper and lower body to provide balanced development. You should also spend at least 15 minutes stretching three times a week, focusing on the lower back.

How many reps?

Do 12–15 reps per set with 30–60 seconds' rest in between sets.

How much weight?

Choose a light-moderate weight that will make the last one or two reps challenging.

How slowly?

Count two seconds up, three seconds down.

How many sets?

Do two or three sets of each exercise.

How much rest between workouts?

Weight train two or three times a week with at least a day's rest in between.

In-season guidelines

As the competitive season approaches, reduce the number of weight training sessions to twice a week and increase time spent in the saddle.

Increase the number of reps and reduce the weights.

THE MARTIAL ARTIST'S WORKOUT

Goal

Martial artists require strength, explosive power and speed as well as endurance. This workout

Muscle group	Exercise	Sets	Reps
Table 21.8	**Martial artist's workout**		
Workout 1 (lower body, back)			
Lower body	Jump-squat	3	8–10
Quadriceps	Leg extension	2	8–10
Hamstrings	Seated leg curl	2	8–10
Calves	Standing calf raise	3	8–10
Back	Pull-up/chin-up	3	8–10
	One-arm dumbbell row	2	8–10
Lower back	Back extension	2	8–10
Abdominals	Exercise ball crunch	2	12–15
	Side bridge	2	Hold for 5 s, repeat five times
Workout 2 (chest, shoulders, arms)			
Chest	Bench press	3	8–10
	Incline dumbbell press	3	8–10
Shoulders	Dumbbell shoulder press	3	8–10
	Dumbbell lateral raise	3	8–10
Triceps	Lying triceps extension	3	8–10
Biceps	Barbell curl	3	8–10
Abdominals	Oblique crunch	2	12–15
	Exercise ball jack-knife	2	12–15

includes exercises for each muscle group. Perform your exercises in an explosive manner, focusing on lifting the weight (i.e. the concentric part of the movement) as fast as possible.

How many reps?

Eight to ten reps per set with 60–90 seconds' rest in between sets.

How much weight?

Select a moderate-heavy weight that will make the last one or two reps challenging.

How slowly?

Press the weight up explosively, one to two seconds down.

How many sets?

Do two or three sets of each exercise.

How much rest between workouts?

Weight train three times a week with at least a day's rest in between, alternating workout 1 (lower body) and workout 2 (upper body).

Table 21.9	Tennis player's workout		
Muscle group	**Exercise**	**Sets**	**Reps**
Shoulders	Overhead press machine	3	10–12
Back	Dumbbell pull-over	3	10–12
Shoulders	Cable lateral raise	3	10–12
Back	Seated cable row	3	10–12
Chest	Pec-deck flye	3	10–12
Legs	Front or reverse lunge	3	10–12
Lower back	Back extension	2	12–15
Calves	Standing calf raise	3	12–15
Abdominals	Exercise ball crunch	2	12–15
	Alternate twisting exercise ball crunch	2	12–15

In-season guidelines

As the competitive season approaches, reduce the number of weight training sessions to twice a week and increase the time spent on sport-specific training.

Reduce the number of sets per body part and increase the number of repetitions to 12–15 to emphasise muscle endurance.

Include plyometric and jump exercises after a good warm-up then follow with strength exercises. Do approximately 10 reps per set with a three- to five-minute rest between sets.

THE TENNIS PLAYER'S WORKOUT

Goal

This workout will increase your muscular endurance and develop some strength. It includes exercises for both the upper and lower body, but focuses on exercises for the shoulders and back.

How many reps?

Do 10–12 reps per set with 60–90 seconds' rest in between sets.

How much weight?

Choose a moderate weight that will make the last one or two reps challenging.

How slowly?

Count two seconds up, three seconds down.

How many sets?

Do three sets of each exercise.

How much rest between workouts?

Weight train two times a week with at least two days' rest in between.

In-season guidelines

As the competitive season approaches, increase the number of reps to 15–20 and reduce the weights.

Spend more time doing sport-specific training.

THE CARDIOVASCULAR PROGRAMME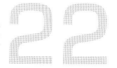

It is not possible to build muscle and lose fat simultaneously. But, over time, you can increase your muscle mass and cut fat gradually. The key is to incorporate cardiovascular exercise training in your weight training programme and pay careful attention to your diet.

Cardiovascular exercise not only burns calories while you are working out but also increases your body's ability to burn fat the rest of the time. Contrary to popular belief, cardiovascular exercise is not counterproductive to a weight training programme. It will not burn hard-earned muscle nor prevent gains in muscle size. In fact, cardiovascular training is essential for any fitness or sports training programme, not just for fat burning but also for its performance- and immunity-boosting effects.

THE BENEFITS OF CARDIO-VASCULAR TRAINING

Cardiovascular training:
- reduces body fat and maintains a low body fat percentage
- increases the body's fat-burning capacity during exercise and rest
- improves body composition
- increases the metabolic rate
- reduces stress and anxiety
- improves confidence, self-esteem and mood
- reduces blood pressure, blood cholesterol and the risk of heart disease
- boosts the immune system.

The science bit...

Regular cardiovascular training increases the body's ability to break down fat by increasing the production of hormone-dependent lipase. This enzyme breaks down fat into its component fatty acids, which are then transported in the bloodstream to the muscles, where they can be broken down to release energy. The better conditioned you are, the higher your levels of fat-burning enzymes and so the more fat you can burn at rest or during exercise. Just as you can train your muscles to become stronger and bigger, so you can train your aerobic system to burn fat more efficiently.

The benefits of cardiovascular training don't end with your workout. Following exercise, your metabolic rate remains elevated for some time as your body replenishes its energy systems. This 'excess post-exercise oxygen consumption' (EPOC) is fuelled almost entirely by fat. Following low-intensity training, the EPOC is very small but following high-intensity training it may be quite large.

Q & A

Which activity?
Any of the following activities may be included in your cardiovascular programme:
- running/treadmill
- fitness/power walking
- stepping machine/stair climber
- cycling/stationary bicycle

- swimming
- aerobic classes/aqua aerobics/step aerobics
- climbing machine
- elliptical training machine
- rowing machine.

The choice depends on your personal preference, and the equipment and time available to you. It's important to plan your workouts around activities that you enjoy, and also to vary the exercise mode as far as possible. The more enthusiastic you are about an activity, the more likely you are to work hard and keep it up. In fact, frequently changing the mode of cardio may produce better results than simply increasing the duration of time you spend doing it as your body becomes more efficient in performing a movement over time, using less energy.

How much and how often?

For optimum cardiovascular fitness and fat-burning, aim for 20–40 minutes, three to five times a week.

How intense?

The harder you train the more calories you burn. As a guide you should be working within your target heart rate zone (THR), which is between 60 and 85% of your maximum heart rate (MHR).[1] Your MHR is the highest heart rate value you can achieve in an all-out effort to the point of exhaustion. It remains constant from day to day and decreases only slightly from year to year – by about one beat per year beginning at 10–15 years of age.

To estimate your MHR, subtract your age from 220. For example, if you were 30, your MHR would be estimated at 190 beats per minute (bpm):

MHR = 220 − 30 = 190 beats per minute
THR zone = (60% x 190) − (85% x 190)
  = 114–162 beats per minute

So, in training, the 30 year old in the example above should aim to keep their heart rate above 114 bpm but below 162 bpm (your lower and upper figures will, of course, depend on using your own age in the above calculation). If you train above your THR zone you begin to work anaerobically and your body can't keep up with the demand for oxygen. You won't be able to sustain this workout intensity very long and will soon reach fatigue. Work within your THR zone to get maximum cardiovascular benefit from your workout.

Whether you choose a high- or low-intensity cardiovascular programme depends on your goals, fitness level and time available. Both types will develop cardiovascular fitness and burn fat but high-intensity exercise (over 70 per cent of your MHR) is more efficient. If time is at a premium, shorter periods of high-intensity exercise will give you the same results in terms of fat loss

The fat-burning zone myth

It's a long-held belief that low-intensity cardiovascular exercise – equivalent to brisk walking or jogging – is the best way to burn fat. It is based on the observation that low-intensity exercise burns a greater percentage of calories from fat than from carbohydrate.[2] In fact, the body burns more fat (as opposed to percentage fat in the fuel mixture) during higher-intensity cardiovascular exercise because the rate of calorie expenditure is higher. It is not the proportion of each fuel metabolised but the total calorie expenditure that is most important. For example, walking (low-intensity cardio) for 60 minutes will burn about 270 kcal, of which approximately 60 per cent (160 kcal) come from fat, while jogging (high-intensity cardio) for 60 minutes will burn about 680 kcal, of which approximately 40 per cent (270 kcal) come from fat. Thus, the higher-intensity exercise results in a greater fat loss over the same workout time.

as longer periods of low-intensity cardio. Training at the lower end of the THR zone is better for beginners and is certainly more attractive for many casual exercisers.

How should I monitor my heart rate?

The best way to monitor your heart rate during your workout is to use a heart rate monitor or take your pulse manually. You can also use the rate of perceived exertion (RPE) scale. This is a subjective rating of how hard you feel you are exercising. The most popular version of this is the Borg scale, a modified version of which is shown in Table 22.1. This 10-point scale ranges from 1 (nothing at all) to 10 (maximum effort). Used correctly, it is a very accurate system for monitoring exercise intensity.

Steady pace or intervals?

Steady pace training – keeping your heart rate fairly constant throughout your workout – builds endurance and a good base level of fitness. Interval training – exercising for short periods at a high intensity, interspersed with lower-intensity recovery periods – builds cardiovascular strength and stamina. The heart and lungs are worked harder during this type of training so they will become stronger and, as a result, you become fitter. It is a more effective way of burning fat than steady pace training because it produces a greater 'after burn' or EPOC, and speeds up your metabolic rate for up to 18 hours after your workout.[3] But before you rush into it, you must be aware that this type of training is only suitable for very well-conditioned athletes and should not be attempted by beginners.

Both types of training can easily be applied to any mode of cardiovascular exercise – running, cycling, stationary bike, stepping machine, elliptical trainer or any other cardio machine. During the interval phases, you increase either your speed or the resistance of the machine (e.g. the incline of a treadmill or the resistance ('level') setting on a stationary bike) in order to reach the required RPE level of 8–9 or 80–90 per cent

Table 22.1	Rating of perceived exertion (RPE)		
At rest		1	Non-exercise HR*
Light activity – sitting working		2	Non-exercise HR
Light activity – walking at leisurely pace		3	Non-exercise HR
Moderate activity – purposeful walking		4	Non-exercise HR
Moderate activity – brisk walking		5	Non-exercise HR
Somewhat hard activity – jogging		6	60% MHR**
Hard activity – running, breathing harder		7	65–75% MHR
Very hard activity – running, conversation just possible		8	80% MHR
Very very hard activity – fast running, conversation difficult		9	85% MHR
Maximum effort – unable to speak		10	MHR
* heart rate			
** maximum heart rate			

MHR. This is maintained for 15 seconds to three minutes, depending on the intensity, followed by a recovery period at an RPE of 4 (somewhat hard) or 60 per cent MHR for 30 seconds to three minutes.

Too much cardio?

More isn't always better, as excessive cardiovascular exercise can result in muscle breakdown and a loss of muscle size and strength. During cardiovascular training, protein can be used for energy, although the misconception that it significantly depletes muscle mass relates more directly to poor diet. An inadequate calorie intake together with high-volume cardiovascular training can result in significant muscle breakdown.

This is induced by the release of the catabolic hormone cortisol (released during all types of high-intensity activity), which outstrips the production of anabolic hormones such as testosterone. Under these conditions there is a net catabolism, or breakdown, of muscle tissue. One study measured a decrease in the size of FT fibres following a three-month period of aerobic training on a treadmill.[4] This may help explain the low muscle mass of many endurance runners.

Dieters who go overboard with cardiovascular training don't realise that a large proportion of their weight loss may be due to muscle loss. When the body doesn't get enough calories it draws upon its reserves, mainly in the form of fat but also from protein, which is found in muscle. You can end up literally cannibalising your own muscle tissue to help your body meet its energy needs. That's the last thing a strength trainer wants.

For this reason cardio should be done in moderation, as per the guidelines above. Moderate amounts of cardio will help you lose fat, and give you numerous health benefits.

High-intensity cardiovascular exercise – this is generally accepted as an intensity corresponding to more than 75 per cent MHR.
Low-intensity cardiovascular exercise – this is generally accepted as an intensity corresponding to less than 75 per cent MHR.

What is the best time for cardiovascular training?

This depends on your individual lifestyle. Choose a time of day that fits in well with your daily schedule; that way you will be less likely to miss a workout. Research suggests that it may be better to perform your cardio and strength training as separate sessions to minimise catabolism (the breakdown of lean mass),[5] but if you prefer to do both in one session complete your weight training workout first when glycogen stores are high. Performing cardio prior to your strength training workout may be counterproductive, resulting in reduced strength and early fatigue due to muscle glycogen depletion.

Weight training burns fat too

It's not only cardio that burns body fat – weight training will also help you get lean.[6] Researchers at Colorado State University measured the RMR of volunteers following an hour's strenuous weight training and discovered that their RMRs remained significantly elevated for three hours after the workout. Even after 16 hours the RMR remained a little higher than normal, as did the rate of fat oxidation. Since RMR makes up the major proportion (60–70 per cent) of total daily energy expenditure, any increase in RMR would have a big impact on your daily calorie output. Therefore, regular strenuous weight training workouts are a very effective strategy for upping calorie burning and losing fat.

STEADY-PACE CARDIOVASCULAR WORKOUT 1

Workout time: 30–50 min (including warm-up and cool-down)
THR zone: 60–75 per cent MHR
RPE: 6–7 (moderate)

This workout is suitable for beginners. Start with a five-minute warm-up, then gradually build up your pace or machine resistance until you reach your training zone (60–75 per cent MHR) or an RPE of 6–7 (moderate). Maintain your intensity in this zone for 20–40 minutes, depending on your fitness and time available. Gradually reduce your pace or resistance for a five-minute cool-down before stretching out.

STEADY-PACE CARDIOVASCULAR WORKOUT 2

Workout time: 30–50 min (including warm-up and cool-down)
THR zone: 75–85 per cent MHR
RPE: 8 (hard–very hard)

This workout is suitable for well-conditioned trainers only. Start with a five-minute warm-up, then gradually build up your pace or machine resistance until you reach your training zone (75–85 per cent MHR) or an RPE of 8 (hard or very hard). Maintain your intensity in this zone for 20–40 minutes. Gradually reduce your pace or resistance for a five-minute cool-down before stretching out.

INTERVAL TRAINING CARDIOVASCULAR WORKOUT

Workout time: 30–50 min (including warm-up and cool-down)
THR zone: 80–90 per cent MHR for high-intensity intervals; 60–65 per cent MHR for low-intensity intervals
RPE: 8–9 (very hard) for high-intensity intervals; 6 (somewhat hard) for low-intensity intervals

This workout is suitable for very well-conditioned trainers only but is a very efficient way to burn fat. Start with a five-minute warm-up, then perform nine sets of two-minute intervals. Adjust your pace or machine resistance to reach your training zone (80–90 per cent MHR) or an RPE of 8–9 for one minute, followed by one or two minutes at 60–65 per cent MHR or an RPE of 6. Gradually reduce your pace or resistance for a five-minute cool-down before stretching out.

SUMMARY OF KEY POINTS

- It is important to include cardio training in a strength training programme to improve body composition, increase the RMR and improve cardiovascular fitness.
- Cardiovascular fitness is developed by performing three to five cardiovascular training sessions lasting 20–40 minutes per week.
- High-intensity cardiovascular exercise is more effective than low-intensity cardiovascular exercise for burning body fat and developing cardiovascular fitness.
- Interval training is more effective than steady pace training for developing cardiovascular fitness.
- Excessive cardiovascular exercise with an inadequate calorie intake, can result in muscle breakdown and loss of muscle mass.

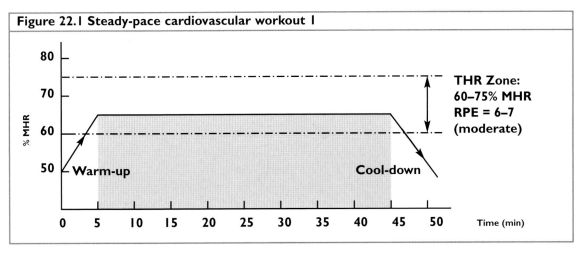

Figure 22.1 Steady-pace cardiovascular workout 1

THR Zone:
60–75% MHR
RPE = 6–7
(moderate)

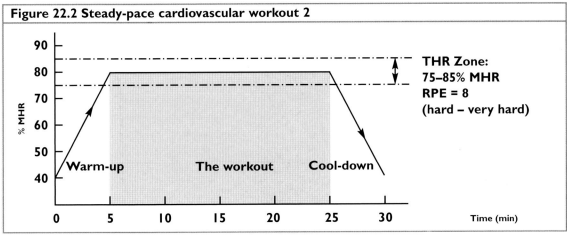

Figure 22.2 Steady-pace cardiovascular workout 2

THR Zone:
75–85% MHR
RPE = 8
(hard – very hard)

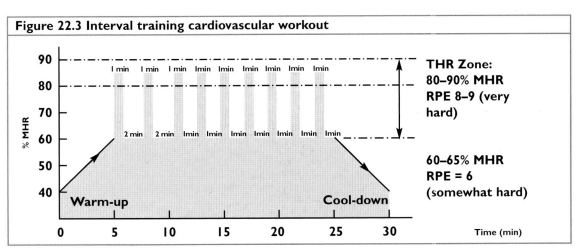

Figure 22.3 Interval training cardiovascular workout

THR Zone:
80–90% MHR
RPE 8–9 (very
hard)

60–65% MHR
RPE = 6
(somewhat hard)

RE-SCULPTING YOUR BODY

You cannot change your basic shape, which is determined by your genes, but with weight training you can refine your dimensions and develop your physique to its best potential.

This chapter shows you how to re-sculpt your body through specific training programmes. Whether you are naturally thin or stocky, you can improve your shape by following the training guidelines for your body type and for specific body parts.

BODY TYPES

The Sheldon system classifies body types into three basic categories:
1. ectomorph
2. mesomorph

3. endomorph.

Most people are a mixture of these three types but tend to resemble one type more strongly. For example, you may share most of the characteristics of a mesomorph (wide shoulders and narrow hips) but have slight endomorphic tendencies as well (gain fat readily).

The ectomorph is lean and thin with little muscle bulk and low body-fat levels. This person has narrow shoulders and hips, and a fast metabolism, which makes it difficult to gain muscle or fat. At the other end of the spectrum, the endomorph has a naturally stocky, rounded build with wide shoulders and wide hips. This person has an even distribution of fat and gains both muscle and fat easily, making training gains less visible. The mesomorph has a naturally athletic build with wide shoulders and

Figure 23.1 Sheldon body types. Mesomorph (left); endomorph (centre); ectomorph (right).

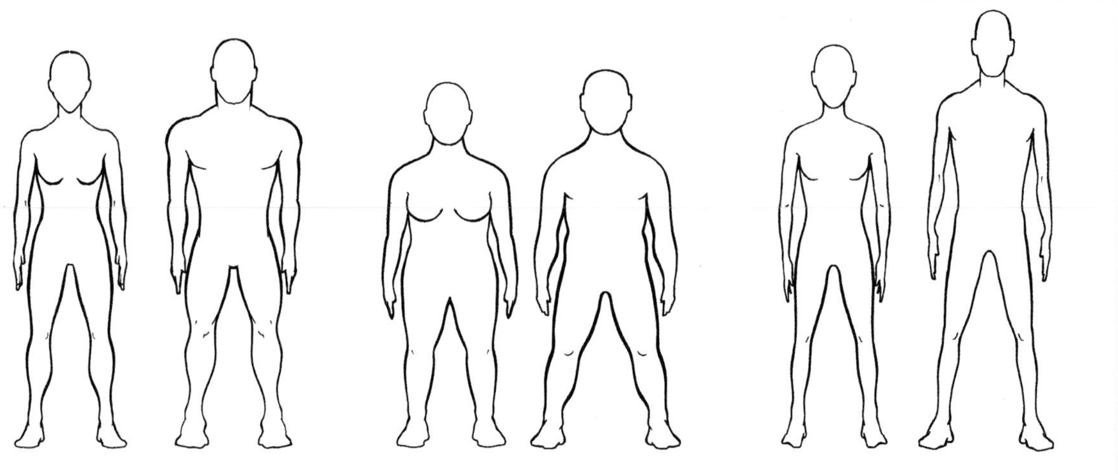

narrow hips. This person gains muscle readily and finds it easy to shed fat, so tends to make the best bodybuilder.

How should an ectomorph train?

If you are an ectomorph, your muscle gains will be slower than those of the other body types. Realistically, you cannot expect to gain much more than 0.5 kg/month, although you may gain muscle faster during the first three to six months. However, don't be discouraged if your gains come slowly – the beginner's programme (pp. 158–63) will help you develop a good foundation of strength. Progress to the intermediate's programme (pp. 164–8) to increase muscle size and strength, concentrating on basic compound movements such as squats, bench presses and dead lifts. These exercises will stimulate larger amounts of muscle mass and a greater number of muscle fibres. Keep isolation exercises to a minimum, and limit your cardiovascular training to two sessions/week, opting for low-intensity rather than high-intensity training (see pp. 195–6). Also follow the weight-gain eating tips (p. 16).

How should an endomorph train?

Endomorphs are naturally strong and generally have little trouble gaining muscle and strength. However, your gains may be hidden under a layer of fat, so the main focus of your training programme should be fat-burning cardiovascular activity. Aim to perform a cardiovascular workout three to six days/week, including at least two high-intensity interval workouts (see p. 196) in addition to your strength training. High-intensity cardiovascular training burns more fat than low-intensity training both during your workout and afterwards. If you do your cardio workout first thing in the morning, your muscles will also burn more calories from fat

(see p. 25). Another way to encourage fat being used for fuel is to avoid eating carbohydrate shortly before your workouts in order to keep insulin levels in your bloodstream low (see p. 25). Following your workouts, wait one hour before eating in order to encourage more fat to be broken down to replenish short-term energy stores. Follow the beginner's programme (see pp. 158–63), to increase muscular endurance and muscle tone – this will give you a good base of strength and a lower body-fat percentage. As your fitness improves, increase the number of circuits, sets and repetitions – this will burn more calories.

How should a mesomorph train?

As a mesomorph, you tend to get good gains from just about anything you do in the gym. However, that's not to say that you can train mindlessly. A well-designed programme will keep you focused and optimise your gains. The key is to use a periodised programme, breaking your training into shorter cycles to achieve year-round gains in strength and size (see pp. 178–82). This will help you avoid overtraining. You should vary your routines frequently, using advanced training techniques such as supersets and descending sets once you have sufficient experience. Change the order of your exercises, the number of sets and repetitions, and the rest intervals used to provide plenty of variety and increase your motivation. Your workout can include a mixture of compound and isolation exercises, and should include cardio training three times per week to keep your body-fat levels low and improve your cardiovascular fitness. Follow the beginner's and intermediate's programmes (see pp. 158–63 and pp. 164–8) progressing to the advanced workouts (see pp. 169–75) once you have at least one year's training experience.

WHAT IS MY OPTIMAL BODY-FAT PERCENTAGE?

It is impossible to set an optimal body-fat percentage that applies to everyone. The body-fat level that your body comfortably reaches without strict dieting is dependent on your genetic make-up as well as your diet and activity. Your natural body type dictates to some extent how much fat you carry and how readily you store it. For example, if you are an ectomorph or mesomorph, you are naturally lean and will be able to achieve a lower body-fat percentage than an endomorph who stores fat easily. But, whatever your natural body type, you can still achieve a lower body-fat level and more defined physique through consistent hard training and healthy eating. The important point is to decide on a level that is realistic for your build and shape.

How low can I go?

Healthy ranges for the general population are 18–25 per cent for women and 13–18 per cent for men.[1] But if you are a strength trainer or bodybuilder, you may desire lower levels. Between 10 per cent and 20 per cent for women and between 6 per cent and 15 per cent for men are common among well-trained athletes – levels that are generally associated with peak performance – but these percentages should be regarded with some caution. If you try to attain a low body-fat percentage that is unnatural for your genetic make-up, you may encounter problems.

For women, a body-fat percentage that is under their individual threshold for menstruation (14–20 per cent) can be risky. Below this, a deficiency of oestrogen and progesterone similar to those levels experienced during and after the menopause can result in amenorrhoea (cessation of menstruation). This can lead to infertility, loss of bone density, stress fractures and premature osteoporosis. Most experts therefore recommend a lower limit of 14 per cent body fat for women.[2]

If a man's body-fat percentage dips too low, there are health risks too. Studies have shown that when men reach a body-fat level of 4–6 per cent, their bodies start to feed on muscle tissue as a source of energy and to allow them to maintain their fat stores at a minimal level.[3] It is definitely unwise, if not impossible, to reduce your body fat below this level. Other studies have found that testosterone levels plummet below 5 per cent body fat, causing reduced sexual drive and fertility.[4]

LEG CLINIC

Symmetry problem: thin legs and difficulty gaining size

Skinny legs produce an overall weak appearance. The symmetry problem is exacerbated if you have a well-developed upper body – a particularly common fault in men who put more emphasis on training their chest, shoulders and arms but neglect to train their legs!

THE SOLUTION

You can increase muscle mass in the leg area by concentrating on compound exercises, which cause maximum stimulation of the FT muscle fibres: squats, dead lifts and leg presses. These are, admittedly, harder to perform than isolation exercises such as leg extensions and curls (which should be avoided) as they require a great deal of physical and mental effort. However, they will produce faster and better results. Perform three to four sets per exercise for six to ten repetitions, using heavy weights that allow you to reach failure.

SYMMETRY PROGRAMME FOR THIN LEGS

Exercise	Sets	Reps
Squat	3–4	6–10
Dead lift	3–4	6–10
Leg press	3–4	6–10

Symmetry problem: lack of hamstring development relative to quadriceps

The back of your thigh appears straight and flat when viewed from the side as it is underdeveloped compared with the quadriceps. This imbalance is a common problem in long/middle-distance cyclists and runners as these activities stress the quadriceps more than the hamstrings. It is also seen in weight trainers who have concentrated on exercising the quadriceps and neglected to balance their leg programme with hamstring exercises.

THE SOLUTION

The imbalance can be corrected by cutting back on quadriceps isolation exercises such as leg extensions, and by including more exercises for the hamstrings, such as leg curls and straight-leg dead lifts. Use relatively heavy weights and keep the reps in the six to ten range. All-round mass-builders such as squats and leg presses should still be included as they stimulate all the leg muscles equally.

SYMMETRY PROGRAMME FOR HAMSTRINGS

Exercise	Sets	Reps
Squat or leg press	3–4	6–10
Straight-leg dead lift	3–4	6–10
Lying or seated leg curl	3–4	6–10

Symmetry problem: fat thighs

Fat thighs are more common in women than men, partly due to hormonal influences (oestrogen and progesterone favour fat deposition in the upper thighs and hips) and partly due to lifestyle. Eating more calories than you need and under-exercising over a period of time cause an increase in body-fat stores. The only way to reduce fat is to combine increased aerobic exercise with a lower-calorie/fat diet. Creams, massage, body brushes or 'detox' supplements cannot remove fat or cellulite.

THE SOLUTION

The solution for fat thighs is to include both strength and aerobic (cardio) exercise in your programme, and reduce the fat content of your diet. Aim for a minimum of 20 minutes' cardio training three to five times a week, gradually increasing this to 45 minutes as you get fitter (see pp. 194–8).

SYMMETRY PROGRAMME FOR FAT THIGHS

Exercise	Sets	Reps
Squat or leg press	2–3	12–15
Front or rear lunge	2–3	12–15
Lying or seated leg curl	2–3	12–15

Symmetry problem: shapeless legs

Although you may have good strength in your legs, they may lack shape. Viewed from the front, your legs make a straight line from the hips to the knees, with no obvious outer sweep to the thigh. From the side, your legs also look straight and neither the quadriceps nor hamstrings make an aesthetic arc. This is due mainly to a lack of muscle development, a symmetry problem common among long-distance runners and people who exercise regularly but relatively infrequently (e.g. once a week).

THE SOLUTION

Your programme should include a combination of compound exercises such as squats, and isolation exercises such as lunges and leg extensions to stimulate overall development. Use moderate to heavy weights and a mixture of low and high repetitions (eight to fifteen).

SYMMETRY PROGRAMME FOR SHAPELESS LEGS

Exercise	Sets	Reps
Squat or leg press	2	8–15
Front or rear lunge	2	8–15
Lying or seated leg curl	2	8–15
Leg extension	2	8–15

Symmetry problem: small calves

Small calves are partly due to genetics and part-ly due to lack of direct calf work. Some people have naturally thin calves due to a high percent-age of ST fibres. This means they have a low capacity for growth and are better suited to endurance work. It is a common mistake to neg-lect calf training, however. Many weight trainers leave them to the end of their workout, when they are tired, and perform little work on them.

THE SOLUTION

If you have naturally thin calves you need to per-form exercises that stress the small percentage of FT that you have there. Unfortunately, everyday activities such as walking and running work only the ST endurance fibres and provide minimal stimulation for growth. Therefore, your pro-gramme should include more emphasis on calf exercises. Perform six to ten sets of eight to twelve repetitions using heavy weights.

SYMMETRY PROGRAMME FOR SMALL CALVES

Exercise	Sets	Reps
Standing calf raise	2–4	8–12
Leg press machine calf press	2–4	8–12
Dumbbell calf raise	2–4	8–12

Symmetry problem: bulky calves

Bulky calves are usually due to the genetic endowment of a high percentage of FT fibres coupled with previous participation in sports such as sprinting, rugby, football and step aero-bics. If you have a high percentage of FT fibres, your calves respond readily to any type of high-intensity exercise.

THE SOLUTION

The only way to reduce the size of a muscle is to stop training it and allow it to atrophy (waste away). Realistically, you should minimise the amount of direct calf work you perform. They will receive sufficient stimulation from everyday activities, such as walking and running, your leg training and any sports that you play.

BACK CLINIC

Symmetry problem: narrow back

Viewed from behind, your torso is straight, nar-row and lacks a pleasing 'V' taper. This is main-ly due to the underdevelopment of the back muscles and is a very common problem, espe-cially in people who do little exercise. It is also seen in long-distance runners, joggers, cyclists, aerobics participants, and many other sports-men, since relatively few sports and activities work this muscle group.

THE SOLUTION

You can build and develop the muscles of the upper and mid-back using heavy compound exercises, such as chins and rowing movements. Perform three to four sets of each exercise for six to ten repetitions. The exercises in this pro-gramme build both width and thickness.

SYMMETRY PROGRAMME FOR A NARROW BACK

Exercise	Sets	Reps
Chins	3–4	6–10
Bent-over barbell row or one-arm row	3–4	6–10
Seated cable row	3–4	6–10

Symmetry problem: weak lower back

The muscles of your lower back, the spinal erectors, are easily overstretched and weakened through poor posture, bearing uneven and heavy loads, sudden twisting, poor exercise technique and lack of direct exercise. This leaves you prone to injury and back pain.

THE SOLUTION

The lower-back muscles can be strengthened by specific exercises, but also by practising safe training techniques during exercises such as the squat and dead lift, which place considerable stress on this area. By holding the abdominals taut during these exercises – indeed during all exercises – you will help avoid injury and strain to the lower back muscles. Include three to four sets of back extensions performed for 10–15 repetitions twice a week with your abdominal routine.

You should also strengthen your abdominal muscles – in particular, the deep (core) muscles in the abdomen and near the lower spine. Perform back extensions and abdominal exercises with the Swiss ball (exercise ball).

SYMMETRY PROGRAMME FOR A WEAK BACK

Exercise	Sets	Reps
Back extension with Swiss ball	2–3	8–12
Crunch with Swiss ball	2–3	8–12

CHEST CLINIC

Symmetry problem: narrow chest

A narrow chest has a straight appearance and makes the shoulders appear rounded and dominating. Viewed from the side it appears flat or even hollow. The width and circumference of your chest depends partly on your bone structure, in particular the size and shape of your rib cage and your clavicles (collarbones), and the size of your pectoral muscles.

THE SOLUTION

A narrow chest can be improved by building up the pectorals and stretching the muscles between the ribs (serratus and intercostals). Poor posture can also exacerbate the symmetry problem, making the chest appear concave. This programme is designed to develop the pectorals. You should use maximum ROM, particularly for the isolation exercises, and perform chest stretches between exercises to improve the flexibility of the pectorals and muscles of the rib cage. Perform two to three sets per exercise for six to ten repetitions.

SYMMETRY PROGRAMME FOR A NARROW CHEST

Exercise	Sets	Reps
Barbell or dumbbell bench press (wide grip)	2–3	6–10
Incline barbell or dumbbell press	2–3	6–10
Dumbbell flye or cable cross-over	2–3	6–10

Symmetry problem: flat upper chest

Viewed from the side, the upper part of your chest appears flat or concave and lacks a pleasing aesthetic curve from your clavicles (collarbones). This symmetry problem is very common, particularly in women who have dieted, since the upper pectorals easily atrophy when calorie and protein intake is reduced over a period of time. A concave upper chest is due to underdevelopment of the upper portion of the pectorals.

THE SOLUTION

Building the upper chest muscles corrects this problem and creates a fuller, more symmetrical chest. It also adds cleavage! Perform all pressing and flye movements on an incline bench set at 30–45°. Use moderate-heavy weights, and perform two to three sets of six to ten repetitions.

SYMMETRY PROGRAMME FOR A FLAT UPPER CHEST

Exercise	Sets	Reps
Incline bench press	2–3	6–10
Incline dumbbell press	2–3	6–10
Incline dumbbell flye	2–3	6–10

SHOULDER CLINIC

Symmetry problem: narrow shoulders

Narrow shoulders greatly affect your total body symmetry. In women, narrow, underdeveloped deltoids accentuate a pear shape, making the hips appear wider than they actually are. In men, they make the whole body look weak and undeveloped, or detract from an otherwise athletic physique. Sometimes, the medial (outer) head is poorly developed relative to the anterior (front) head. This is common in weight trainers that focus on chest exercises such as the bench press at the expense of shoulder exercises.

The width of your shoulders is determined partly by the length of your clavicles (collarbones) and partly by the amount of muscle mass development. Obviously, you cannot change the former but you can significantly increase the width of your shoulders and greatly improve your overall body symmetry by developing your deltoids. The medial head is mostly responsible for creating width but all three heads need to be developed equally to create good symmetry and avoid injury.

THE SOLUTION

To widen the shoulders you need to build up the muscle mass by focusing on compound exercises such as shoulder presses and upright rows. These place the greatest stimulus on the shoulders and therefore lead to fastest gains in size and strength. You should also include lateral raises, as these work the medial head directly and create width. Perform three to four sets of six to ten repetitions of each exercise, using heavy weights for the pressing movements.

SYMMETRY PROGRAMME FOR NARROW SHOULDERS

Exercise	Sets	Reps
Dumbbell press	3–4	6–10
Upright row	3–4	6–10
Lateral raise	3–4	6–10

Symmetry problem: rounded shoulders

Rounded shoulders are the result of poor posture, bad sitting position, poor muscle strength in the upper back and lack of flexibility in the chest muscles. Viewed from the side, your head juts forwards, your upper back is rounded, your rib cage is reduced, or even hollowed, and your shoulders droop. It is one of the most common postural faults in men and women. Rounded shoulders are also common in weight trainers who have overly developed the anterior head of the deltoids relative to the posterior head. Thus, the anterior head receives a disproportionate amount of stress compared with the medial and posterior heads, creating muscular imbalance.

THE SOLUTION

Strengthening the trapezius and muscles of the upper back will pull the shoulders back into correct alignment. Increasing the flexibility of your chest muscles will expand the rib cage and allow the shoulders to move back easily into alignment. You should also strengthen the deltoids, especially the posterior head, which will help correct any muscular imbalance. Perform three sets of eight to twelve repetitions of each exercise using a moderate weight.

SYMMETRY PROGRAMME FOR ROUNDED SHOULDERS

Exercise	Sets	Reps
Upright row	2–3	8–12
Bent-over lateral raise	2–3	8–12
Shrug	2–3	8–12
Shoulder press	2–3	8–12

ARM CLINIC

Symmetry problem: skinny arms

Poorly muscled arms are the result of a lack of direct biceps and triceps exercise. Your muscles are small and underdeveloped, lack density, and appear straight and flat with no discernible shape.

THE SOLUTION

The problem can easily be corrected by including mass-building exercises for your arm muscles, such as barbell curls, triceps extensions and triceps push-downs. These movements recruit the largest number of muscle fibres and therefore place maximum stress on the muscles, producing the fastest gains in size and strength.

Your programme should include more triceps work than biceps work because the triceps provide a much greater proportion of the upper-arm muscle mass than the biceps (see pp. 94–5). (Many weight trainers make the mistake of overtraining their biceps and neglecting their triceps in an attempt to get bigger arms.) Select a total of four to six sets for your biceps, and six to nine

sets for your triceps, performing six to ten repetitions per set with a heavy weight.

SYMMETRY PROGRAMME FOR SKINNY ARMS

Exercise	Sets	Reps
Barbell curl	2–3	6–10
Preacher curl	2–3	6–10
Lying triceps extension	2–3	6–10
Triceps press-down	2–3	6–10
Bench dip	2–3	6–10

Symmetry problem: bulky, shapeless arms

Viewed from the side, your arms appear chunky, straight and lacking in definition. You have developed good muscle mass in them but there is no real peak to the biceps, nor a discernible horseshoe outline to the triceps. This problem is partly due to excessive subcutaneous fat covering the muscles' outline, and partly due to poor exercise technique, shortening the ROM, which leads to sub-optimal development of the muscle along its whole length.

THE SOLUTION

By reducing your body fat you will reduce the fat layer covering your triceps and biceps, and improve your muscle definition. So include more cardio training (aim for three to five sessions of 20–30 minutes per week) and follow a fat-burning eating plan. The programme includes only one mass-building exercise for biceps and triceps, and two isolation exercises, which place greater demand on different parts of the muscles' length. Ensure that you use the full ROM and do not shorten the motion. Use slightly higher repetitions (up to 15) and moderate weights, and concentrate on the feel of the movement.

SYMMETRY PROGRAMME FOR BULKY ARMS

Exercise	Sets	Reps
Concentration curl	2	10–15
Incline dumbbell curl	2	10–15
Dumbbell preacher curl	2	10–15
One-arm triceps extension	2	10–15
Bench dip	2	10–15
Triceps kickback	2	10–15

ABDOMINAL CLINIC

Symmetry problem: lower tummy bulge

Viewed from the side, the lower part of your tummy appears rounded and protruding. This may be due to one or more of the following:

• poor posture
• poor muscle tone in the lower and deep abdominals
• overstretched abdominals
• an accumulation of fat.

The posture problem – lordosis – is caused by an excessive forward pelvic tilt. The hip flexors (which connect the thigh bone with the lower vertebrae) become tighter, and pull and compress the lower vertebrae, leading to excessive arching in your lower back.

THE SOLUTION

Lordosis can be corrected by retraining the tilt of your pelvis (aim to maintain a neutral tilt), stretching the hip flexors and strengthening the abdominals (especially the lower part of the abdominis rectus and the transverse abdominis). Body fat should be reduced if necessary by increasing aerobic activity (aim for three to five cardio sessions per week of 20–45 minutes), and following a fat-burning eating plan. This programme emphasises the lower part of the rectus abdominis and the transverse abdominis, one of the deeper 'core' muscles (see pp. 107–8) but also

includes exercises for the other abdominal muscles to maintain good overall development. Performing the abdominal exercises using a Swiss ball (exercise ball) will strengthen the core muscles and improve stability (see pp. 138–9). Read the technique notes on p. 108 too.

SYMMETRY PROGRAMME FOR A LOWER TUMMY BULGE

Exercise	Sets	Reps
Reverse crunch	2	10–15
Hanging leg raise	2	10–15
Hip flexor stretch	2*	30–60 s
Plank	1	60–90 s
Exercise ball pull-in	1	10–15

*Perform twice on each leg.

Symmetry problem: wide waist

Viewed from the front, your waist appears wide relative to your hips and chest and your tummy may protrude slightly. This may simply be due to a 'short' waist structure, or to an excess of fat stored at the sides of the waist and poor muscle tone of the obliques.

THE SOLUTION

Fat stored at the sides of the waist cannot be spot-reduced by diet or exercise. However, it can be reduced when overall body-fat levels are reduced through increasing aerobic activity (three to five cardio sessions per week of 20–45 minutes) and following a fat-burning eating plan.

Unfortunately, your basic skeletal structure cannot be changed. A naturally short mid-section is determined by the distance between your ribs and pelvis, and can make the waist appear wider than it actually is. However, you can still improve your appearance by working the abdominal muscles and particularly the obliques. This will create a narrower waistline and better posture. This programme emphasises the internal and external obliques but also includes exercises for the rectus abdominis to maintain good overall development. Performing the abdominal exercises with a Swiss ball (exercise ball) will strengthen the core muscles, i.e. the deeper abdominal muscles and the muscles close to the lower spine and pelvis that improve your stability, coordination and posture (see pp. 138–9).

SYMMETRY PROGRAMME FOR A WIDE WAIST

Exercise	Sets	Reps
Oblique crunch	1–2	10–15
Side crunch	1–2	10–15
Alternate twisting		
Exercise ball crunch	1–2	10–15
Side bridge	1–2	10–15

SUMMARY OF KEY POINTS

- Your personal training programme should be tailored to suit your natural body type, with a different emphasis placed on exercise selection, sets, repetitions, intensity and cardio training.
- Ectomorphs should focus on mass-building, using compound exercises, heavy weights, a high training intensity and limited cardio training.
- Endomorphs require more cardio training to burn fat, and can afford to do more sets and repetitions to increase calorie burning.
- Mesomorphs experience good gains from most programmes but should employ periodisation and plenty of variety to optimise developments and avoid overtraining.
- Your body-fat level depends on your genetic make-up, including your natural body type, as well as diet and activity.
- A body-fat percentage of 6–15 per cent for men and 10–20 per cent for women is generally associated with peak performance.
- A lower limit of 5 per cent for men and 14 per cent for women is recommended. Attaining lower body-fat percentages is associated with oestrogen deficiency in women and testosterone deficiency in men, as well as other health risks.
- Most symmetry problems can be remedied by using the SMART principles of programme design (see pp. 128–30) – selecting specific exercises, performed in a particular order for the right amount of sets and repetitions, and at the correct intensity.

TROUBLESHOOTING

Many trainers fail to make significant progress despite many months or years of training. Initial gains in muscular endurance and muscle tone are relatively rapid in beginners but gains in muscle size and strength can be painstakingly slow after the first six months. To make improvements on a regular basis, you need to look carefully at every aspect of your training programme. This chapter reveals the most common mistakes made in the gym and how to avoid them.

CHOOSING THE WRONG EXERCISES

The selection of exercises in your programme depends on your specific goals and your training experience. For example, if your goal is to increase muscle size, you have to prioritise maximal-stimulation or compound exercises (e.g. squats, bench presses, barbell rows, shoulder presses) in your programme. These stimulate the largest muscles and the greatest proportion of fibres in those muscles. Isolation exercises (e.g. triceps kickbacks, biceps curls), which work smaller muscle groups or a smaller proportion of the muscle fibres in that muscle group, should be kept to a minimum and performed last in your workout.

DOING TOO MANY REPETITIONS

If you can do more than about 12 repetitions, it means that you are using too light a weight to stimulate growth in the FT muscle fibres. Doing more than 12 repetitions will improve muscular endurance but produce only small improvements in strength and size. Therefore, if it is muscle growth you want, select a weight that will allow you to perform six to twelve repetitions. Using a heavier weight that allows you to perform no more than six repetitions will improve your maximum strength. This method will not produce maximum size but can be useful for overcoming training plateaux within a hypertrophy programme.

DOING TOO MANY SETS

Research has established that less is best when it comes to building size and mass. The exact number of sets required to achieve maximal stimulation of the muscle fibres is debatable. The general recommendation for muscle size is eight to twelve sets for larger muscle groups and three to eight for smaller muscle groups, but the most important goal is to achieve overload. Whether you achieve this after one set or twelve is less important.

Advocates of single-set training claim overload can be achieved by performing a strict set of six to ten repetitions with a heavy weight to failure, following a few warm-up sets. Once overload has been achieved, there is no benefit in performing further sets. Doing too many sets also leads to glycogen depletion and increased protein (muscle) breakdown, creating a net catabolic (breakdown) state – just the opposite of your goal! If you can perform more sets than the recommended range, this means you have failed to train hard enough to reach overload and stimulate growth.

NOT ENOUGH REST

If you don't give your body enough rest between workouts, you will not experience gains in mass or strength. One of the biggest mistakes made by beginners in their desire to make rapid gains is training too frequently. It is tempting to think that the more often you train, the faster you will gain mass, but in fact the opposite is true. Growth can only take place after compensation and full recovery. In other words, training before you have fully recovered can lead to a net protein (muscle) breakdown and, over time, can lead to overtraining. As a general guideline, beginners should leave one to three days' recovery between workouts, while experienced weight trainers should leave three to seven days between training the same muscle group due to the greater workout intensity (see p. 144).

LACK OF PROGRESSION

Many weight trainers become disheartened when strength gains slow down or plateau despite maintaining a consistent workout programme. Indeed, it is easy to get stuck in a rut if you use the same weights, same exercises and same number of sets and reps. The muscles can soon adapt to a routine programme if the stimulus remains the same. In order to continue making strength and mass gains your training programme must be progressive. That is, you must continue to increase the amount of stimulus applied. This may be achieved in one of the following ways:

- change the number of reps – either increase them up to a maximum of 12 (for developing

muscle size), or decrease them to three to six, using a heavier weight (for developing maximum strength)
- increase the number of sets – up to a maximum of 12 for major muscle groups and eight for smaller muscle groups
- change the type of exercises you perform and vary your workout – e.g. if you always perform lat pull-downs, seated rows and close-grip chins for your back, change to wide-grip chins, one-arm dumbbell rows and pull-overs
- use different variations of exercises – e.g. different grip distances or foot positions (see the wide range of variations outlined in Chapters 4–9)
- change the order of your exercises – e.g. instead of always working from the largest to the smallest muscle groups, use the pre-exhaustion method for one workout (see p. 138), or try new sequences such as alternating pushing and pulling exercises, or using supersets either for the same muscle group or for opposing muscle groups (see pp. 137–8)
- change the training tempo – e.g. take shorter rest periods between sets
- use advanced training methods – e.g. eccentric training, forced or assisted reps, descending sets or supersets
- change the training split – e.g. train your shoulders and back together instead of your shoulders and arms.

PARTIAL RANGE OF MOVEMENT

If you use an incomplete ROM, the muscle fibres receive only partial stimulation. You may be able to use a heavier weight doing partial repetitions but the overall stimulus applied will be greatly reduced. This is a very common fault made by weight trainers keen to increase the weight lifted – but it is at the expense of correct form. Research has proved that taking a movement to the end of its natural range produces a more powerful anabolic stimulus than exercising over an incomplete ROM. It also produces better muscle shape, and prevents muscle shortening and reduced flexibility. You will therefore achieve considerably greater gains by performing each repetition through its complete ROM, even if it means using a lighter weight.

POOR TECHNIQUE

Many weight trainers sacrifice technique in an attempt to lift heavier weights. Not only does this increase the risk of injury but it limits gains in strength and mass. 'Cheating' movements – such as arching the back and bouncing the bar off the chest when performing a bench press, bending forwards excessively when squatting or swinging backwards when doing barbell curls – reduce the work done by the prime mover muscles and put the back at risk of injury. Correct technique is therefore vital in order to make continued gains in strength and mass.

LACK OF GOAL-SETTING

It is essential to set goals if you want to achieve results (see pp. 128–33). First, be clear about exactly what you want to achieve, setting specif-ic goals (e.g. 'I want to gain 5 kg of muscle') that are measurable and realistic. Second, write down the reasons why you want to change. Third, set a timescale for achieving your goals. Finally, monitor your progress by filling in a training diary. Reward your progress once you reach each mini-goal.

SUMMARY OF KEY POINTS

• Failure to make progress is often due to a combination of reasons centred on programme design, training technique and goal-setting.
• Slow gains may be the result of poor programme design – for example, choosing inappropriate exercises, performing too many repetitions or sets, or taking inadequate rest.
• A lack of programme progression leads to training plateaux as muscles require continual changes in stimulus in order to grow.
• Progression can be achieved by changing any one of the following variables: the number of repetitions and sets; the type and order of exercises; the training tempo and training split.
• Poor technique and incomplete ROM are common faults that will reduce your gains.
• Failure to set specific goals and make a plan of action sets you up for failure.

APPENDIX

Quick Reference for the Major Muscle Groups, their Locations, Main Functions and Exercises

Muscle	Location	Main function	Exercises
Legs			
Quadriceps • Rectus femoris • Vastus lateralis • Vastus medialis • Vastus intermedialus	Front of thigh	Collectively extend the knee. Rectus femoris also flexes the hip	• Squat • Dead lift • Leg press • Leg extension • Front lunge • Reverse lunge • Dumbbell step-ups
Adductors • Adductor brevis • Adductor longus • Adductor magnus	Inner thigh	Pull the legs together	• Squat • Dead lift
Abductors • Gluteus minimus • Gluteus medius	Outer thigh	Pull the legs sideways	• Squat • Dead lift
Hamstrings • Biceps femoris • Semiteninosus • Semimembranosus	Back of thigh	Bend the knee and pull the hip back	• Squat • Dead lift • Leg press • Front lunge • Reverse lunge • Seated leg curl • Straight-leg dead lift • Dumbbell step-ups
Gastrocnemius	Calf	Bends the knee and straightens the ankle	• Standing calf raise • One-legged dumbbell calf raise • Calf press • Seated calf raise

Muscle	Location	Main function	Exercises
Legs cont.			
Soleus	Calf	Straightens the ankle	• Standing calf raise • One-leg dumbbell calf raise • Seated calf raise • Calf press
Gluteals			
Gluteus maximus	Backside	Extends the hip and rotates it outwards	• Squat • Dead lift • Leg press • Front lunge • Reverse lunge • Straight-leg dead lift • Back extension • Dumbbell step-ups
Gluteus medius	Backside	Abducts and rotates the hip inwards	• Squat • Dead lift • Leg press • Front lunge • Reverse lunge • Straight-leg dead lift • Back extension • Dumbbell step-ups
Gluteus minimus	Backside	Stabilises the hip, and abducts and rotates it inwards	• Squat • Dead lift • Leg press • Front lunge • Reverse lunge • Straight-leg dead lift • Back extension • Dumbbell step-ups
Back			
Latissimus dorsi	Upper back	Draws the arms downwards	• Dead lift • Lat pull-down • Pull-up/chin-up • One-arm dumbbell row • Seated cable row • Bent-over barbell row • Straight-arm pull-down • Machine row • Dumbbell pull-over

Muscle	Location	Main function	Exercises
Back cont.			
Trapezius	Upper and mid-back	Draws the shoulder blades backwards	• Dead lift • Pull-up/chin-up • One-arm dumbbell row • Seated cable row • Bent-over barbell row • Straight-arm pull-down • Machine row • Dumbbell shrug • *Dumbell press* • *Lateral raise* • Upright row • *Bent-over lateral raise*
Rhomboids	Deep central upper back	Draws the shoulder blades backwards	• Lat pull-down • Pull-up/chin-up • One-arm dumbbell row • Seated cable row • Bent-over barbell row • Straight-arm pull-down • Machine row • *Dumbell press*
Infraspinatus	Shoulder blades	Rotates the arm outwards	• Pull-up/chin-up • One-arm dumbbell row
Teres major	Shoulder blades	Rotates the arm outwards	• Pull-up/chin-up • One-arm dumbbell row • Seated cable row • Bent-over barbell row • Machine row • Straight-arm pull-down
Teres minor	Shoulder blades	Rotates the arm outwards	• Pull-up/chin-up • One-arm dumbbell row • Seated cable row • Bent-over barbell row • Straight-arm pull-down • Machine row

Muscle	Location	Main function	Exercises
Back cont.			
Erector spinae	Lower back	Flexes the spine and keeps you upright when standing	• Barbell squat • Dead lift • Straight-leg dead lift • Back extension • Back extensions • Dorsal raise • *Seated cable row*
Chest			
Pectoralis major	Chest	Pulls the arm in front of the chest from any position, flexes the shoulder to allow pushing and lifts the arm forwards	• Barbell bench press • Bench press machine • Dumbbell bench press • Dumbbell flye • Pec dec flye • Cable cross-over • Exercise ball press-up/ push-up
Pectoralis minor	Chest	Lowers the shoulder blade	• Incline barbell bench press • Incline dumbbell bench press • Low-pulley cable cross-over
Shoulders			
Anterior deltoids	Shoulder	Lifts arm forwards and upwards	• Dumbbell press • Overhead press machine • Upright row • *Barbell bench press* • *Dumbbell bench press* • *Incline barbell bench press* • *Incline dumbell bench press* • *Dumbbell flye* • *Pee dec flye* • *Cable cross-over* • *Lateral raise*
Medial deltoid	Shoulder	Lifts arm to the side	• Dumbbell press • Lateral raise • Upright row • Overhead press machine

Muscle	Location	Main function	Exercises
Shoulders cont.			
Posterior deltoid	Shoulder	Lifts arm to the rear and draws the elbow backwards	• Bent-over lateral raise • *Lat pull-down* • *Chins* • *One-arm row*
Arms			
Triceps	Outside of the upper arm	Partially or fully straightens the arm from a bent position	• Lying tricep extension • Triceps kickback • Triceps push-down • Reverse-grip triceps push-down • Seated overhead triceps extension • *Barbell bench press* • *Dumbbell bench press* • *Incline barbell bench press* • *Incline dumbbell bench press* • *Dumbbell press* • Bench dip
Biceps brachii	Front of the upper arm	Bends the elbow, rotates the forearm and assists in raising the shoulder forwards	• Barbell curl • Preacher curl • Dumbbell curl • Incline dumbbell curl • Concentration curl • *Lat pull-down* • *Pull-up/chin-up* • *One-arm row* • *Bent-over barbell row* • *Upright row*
Brachialis	Front of the upper arm beneath the biceps	Bends the elbow	• Barbell curl • Preacher curl
Brachioradialis	Top side of forearm	Bends the elbow, rotates the forearm	• *Lat pull-down* • *Chins* • *Seated cable row* • *Bent-over barbell row* • *Upright row* • *Barbell curl* • *Preacher curl* • *Dumbbell curl* • *Incline dumbbell curl*

Muscle	Location	Main function	Exercises
Arms cont.			
Brachioradialis cont.			• *Concentration curl* • *Triceps push-down*
Abdominals			
Obliques – internal and external	Waist	Rotates and flexes the trunk to the side	• Side bridge • Oblique crunch • Side crunch • Alternate twisting exercise-ball crunch
Rectus abdominis	Centre of the abdomen	Flexes the spine	• Crunch • Exercise ball crunch • Reverse crunch • Hanging leg raise • Hip thrust • Side crunch • Exercise-ball pull-in • Plank • Side bridge • Exercise-ball jack-knife
Transversus abdominis	Sheathing the abdomen	Supports the abdomen	• All the abdominal exercise performed with an exercise ball

Note: Exercises in italics indicate those in which the muscles are not the target muscles being developed.

REFERENCES

Chapter 1

1. Campbell, W. *et al.* (1994), 'Increased energy requirements and changes in body composition with resistance training in older adults', *Am. J. Clin Nutr.*, vol. 60, pp. 167–75.

2. Forbes, G. B. (1976), 'The adult decline in lean body mass', *Human Biology*, vol. 48, pp. 161–73.

3. Evans, W. and Rosenberg, I. (1992), *Biomarkers* (New York: Simon & Schuster).

4. Hurley, B. (1994), 'Does strength training improve health status?', *Strength & Cond. J.*, vol. 16, pp. 7–13.

5. Taafe, D. R. *et al.* (1997), 'High impact exercise promotes bone gain in well-trained female athletes', *J. Bone Miner. Res.*, vol. 12 (2), pp. 255–60.

6. Menkes, A. *et al.* (1993), 'Strength training increases regional bone mineral density and bone remodelling in middle-aged and older men', *J. Appl. Physiol.*, vol. 74, pp. 2478–84.

7. Keyes, A. et al. (1973), 'Basal metabolism and age of adult man', Metabolism, vol. 22, pp. 579–87.

8. Westcott, W. (1995), *Strength Fitness: Physiological Principles and Training Techniques*, 4th edn (Dubuque, Iowa: William C. Brown Publishers).

9. Stone, M. *et al.* (1982), 'Physiological effects of a short-term resistance training programme on middle-aged untrained men', *Nat. Strength & Cond. Assoc. J.*, vol. 4, pp. 16–20.

10. Risch, S. *et al.* (1993), 'Lumbar strengthening in low back pain patients', *Spine*, vol. 18, pp. 232–8.

Chapter 2

1. Goldberg, A. L. *et al.* (1975), 'Mechanism of work-induced hypertrophy of skeletal muscle', *Med. Sci. Sports Exerc.*, vol. 7, pp. 248–61.

2. Macdougall, J. D. *et al.* (1994), 'Muscle fibre number in biceps brachii in bodybuilders and control subjects', *J. Appl. Physiol.*, vol. 57, pp. 1399–403.

3. Sale, D. G. *et al.* (1987), 'Voluntary strength and muscle characteristics in untrained men and women and bodybuilders', *J. Appl. Physiol.*, vol. 62, pp. 1786–93.

4. Macdougall, J. D. *et al.* (1979), 'Mitochondrial volume density in human skeletal muscle following heavy resistance training', *Med. Sci. Sports Exerc.*, vol. 11 (20), pp. 164–6.

5. Macdougall, J. D. *et al.* (1980), 'Muscle ultra-structure characteristics of elite powerlifters and bodybuilders', *Med. Sci. Sports Exerc.*, vol. 2, p. 131.

6. Schmidtbleicher, D. and Haralambie, G. (1981), 'Changes in contractile proteins of muscle after strength training in man', *Eur. J. Appl. Physiol.*, vol. 46, pp. 221–8.

7. Dons, B. K. *et al.* (1979), 'The effect of weight lifting exercise related to muscle fibre composition and muscle cross-sectional area in humans', *Eur. J. Appl. Physiol.*, vol. 40, pp. 95–106.

8. Gatorade Sports Science Institute (1995), 'Roundtable on methods of weight gain in athletes', *Sports Science Exchange,* vol. 6 (3), pp. 1–4.

Chapter 3

1. Williams, C. and Devlin, J. T. (eds) (1992), *Foods, Nutrition and Performance: An International Scientific Consensus* (London: Chapman & Hall).

2. Hawley, J. and Burke, L. (1998), 'The training diet', in *Peak Performance,* Chapter 10 (St Leonards, NSW: Allen & Unwin), pp. 211–32.

3. Leeds A. *et al.* (2000), *The Glucose Revolution* (London: Hodder & Stoughton), pp. 215–23.

4. Balon, T. W. *et al.* (1992), 'Effects of carbohydrate loading and weight lifting on muscle girth', *Int. J. Sport Nutr.,* vol. 2, pp. 328–4.

5. Kraemer, W. J. *et al.* (1996) 'Physiological mechanisms of adaptation', *Exerc. Sports Sci. Rev.,* vol. 24, pp. 363–97.

6. Tarnopolsky, M. A. *et al.* (1992) 'Evaluation of protein requirements for trained strength athletes', *J. Appl. Physiol.,* vol. 73, pp. 1986–95.

7. Lemon, P. W. R. (1998), 'Effects of exercise on dietary protein requirements', *Int. J. Sport Nutr.,* vol. 8, pp. 426–47.

8. Simopoulos, A. P. and Robinson, J. (1998), *The Omega Plan* (New York: HarperCollins).

9. Kremer, J. M. (1996), 'Effects of modulation of inflammatory and immune parameters in patients with rheumatis and inflammatory disease receiving dietary supplements of n-3 and n-6 fatty acids', *Lipids,* vol. 31, pp. S243–7.

10. Tsintzas, O. K. et al. (1996), 'Influence of carbohydrate supplementation early in exercise on endurance running capacity', *Med. Sci. Sports Exerc.,* vol. 28, pp. 1373–9.

11. Fahey, T. D. et al. (1993), 'The effects of intermittent liquid meal feeding on selected hormones and substrates during intense weight training', *Int. J. Sport Nutr.,* vol. 3, pp. 67–75.

12. Jeukendrup, A. E. *et al* (1997), 'Carbohydrate–electrolyte feedings improve 1-h time trial cycling performance', *Int. J. Sports Med.,* vol. 18, pp. 125–9.

13. Ivy, J. L. *et al.* (1988), 'Muscle glycogen synthesis after exercise: effect of time on carbohydrate ingestion', *J. Appl. Physiol.,* vol. 64, pp. 1480–5.

14. Baker, S. K. et al. (1994), 'Immediate post-training carbohydrate supplementation improves subsequent performance in trained cyclists', *Sports Med. Training Rehab.,* vol. 5, pp. 131–5.

15. Zawadski, K. M. *et al.* (1992), 'Carbohydrate–protein complex increases the rate of muscle glycogen storage after exercise', *J. Appl. Physiol.,* vol. 72 (5), pp. 1854–9.

16. Ready, S. L. *et al.* (1999) 'The effect of two sports drink formulations on muscle stress and performance', *Med. Sci. Sports Exerc.* Vol. 31 (5), p. S119.

17. Tarnopolsky, M. A. *et al.* (1997) 'Post exercise protein–carbohydrate and carbohydrate supplements increase muscle glycogen in males and females', *J. Appl. Physiol. Abstracts,* vol. 4, p. 332A.

18. Chandler, R. M. *et al.* (1994), 'Dietary supplements affect the anabolic hormones after weight-training exercise', *J. Appl. Physiol.,* vol. 76 (2), pp. 834–9.

19. Bloomer, R. J. *et al.* (2000), 'Alterations in mood following acute post-exercise feeding with variance in macronutrient mix', *Med. Sci. Sports Exerc.,* Supplement, vol. 32 (5), no. 121.

20. ACSM/ADA/DC (2000), 'Position of the American Dietetic Association, Dietitians of Canada, and the American College of Sports Medicine: nutrition and athletic performance', *Med. Sci. Sports Exerc.,* vol. 32 (12), pp. 2130–45.

21. Kleiner, S. M. *et al.* (1994), 'Nutritional status of nationally ranked elite bodybuilders', *Int. J. Sport Nutr.,* vol. 4, pp. 54–69.

22. Newton, L. E. *et al.* (1993), 'Changes in psychological state and self-reported diet during various phases of training in competitive bodybuilders', *J. Strength Cond. Res.,* vol. 7 (3), pp. 153–8.

23. Telford, R. *et al.* (1992) 'The effect of 7–8 months of vitamin/mineral supplementation on athletic performance', *Int. J. Sport Nutr.,* vol. 2, pp. 135–53.

24. Singh, A. *et al.* (1992), 'Chronic multivitamin–mineral supplementation does not enhance physical performance', *Med. Sci. Sport Exerc.,* vol. 24, pp. 726–32.

25. Goldfarb, A. H. (1999), 'Nutritional antioxidants as therapeutic and preventative modalities in exercise-induced muscle damage', *Can. J. Appl. Physiol.,* vol. 24 (3), pp. 249–66.

26. Krotkiewski, M. *et al.* (1994), 'Prevention of muscle soreness by pre-treatment with antioxidants', *Scand. J. Med. Sci. Sports,* vol. 4, pp. 191–9.

27. Hultman, E. *et al.* (1996), 'Muscle creatine loading in man', *J. Appl. Physiol.,* vol. 81, pp. 232–9.

28. Volek, J. S. and Kraemer, W. J. (1996), 'Creatine supplementation: its effect on human muscular performance and body composition', *J. Strength Cond. Res.,* vol. 10 (3), pp. 200–10.

29. Volek, J. S. *et al.* (1996), 'Creatine supplementation enhances muscular performance during high intensity resistance exercise', *J. Amer. Diet. Assoc.,* vol. 97, pp. 765–70.

30. Volek, J. S. *et al.* (1999), 'Performance and muscle fibre adaptations to creatine supplementation and heavy resistance training', *Med. Sci. Sports Exerc.,* vol. 31 (8), pp. 1147–56.

31. Kreider, R. *et al.* (1996), 'Effects of ingesting supplements designed to promote lean tissue accretion on body composition during resistance training', *Int. J. Sport Nutr.,* vol. 63, pp. 234–46.

32. Harris, R. (1998), 'Ergogenics 1', *Peak Performance,* vol. 112 (Dec.), pp. 2–6.

33. Stout, J. *et al.* (1997), 'The effects of a supplement designed to augment creatine uptake on exercise performance and fat-free mass in football players', *Med. Sci. Sports Exerc.,* vol. 29 (5), p. S251.

34. Robinson, T. M. *et al.* (2000), 'Dietary creatine supplementation does not affect some haematological indices, or indices of muscle damage and hepatic and renal function', *Brit. J. Sports. Med.,* vol. 34 (9), pp. 284–8.

35. Nissen, S. *et al.* (1996), 'Effect of leucine metabolite HMB on muscle metabolism during resistance exercise training', *J. Appl. Physiol.,* vol. 81, pp. 2095–104.

36. Nissen, S. L. *et al.* (1997), 'Effect of feeding HMB on body composition and strength in women', *FASEB J.,* vol. 11, p. A150.

37. Slater, G. *et al.* (2001), 'HMB supplementation does not affect changes in strength or body composition during resistance training in trained men', *Int. J. Sport Nutr.,* vol. 11, pp. 383–96.

38. Kreider, R. B. *et al.* (2000), 'Effects of calcium-HMB supplementation during training on markers of catabolism, body composition, strength and sprint performance', *J. Exerc. Physiol.,* vol. 3 (4), pp. 48–59.

39. Castell, L. M. and Newsholme, E. A. (1997), 'The effects of oral glutamine supplementation on athletes after prolonged exhaustive exercise', *Nutrition,* vol. 13 (7), pp. 738–42.

40. Leder, B. Z. *et al.* (2000), 'Oral androstenedione administration and serum testosterone concentrations in young men', *J.A.M.A.,* vol. 283 (6), pp. 779–82.

41. Broeder, C. E. *et al.* (2000), 'The Andro Project: physiological and hormonal influences of androstenedione supplementation in men 35 to 65 years old participating in a high-intensity resistance training program', *Arch. Int. Med.,* vol. 160 (20), pp. 3093–104.

42. Catlin, D. H. *et al.* (2000), 'Trace contamination of over the counter androstenedione and positive urine test results for a nandrolone metabolite', *J.A.M.A.,* vol. 284 (20), pp. 2618–21.

43. Thom, E. (1997), 'Efficacy and tolerability of Tonalin CLA on body composition in

humans', Medstat Research Ltd, presented at the 1997 Federation for Applied Science and Experimental Biology (FASEB) national meeting in New Orleans.

44. Ferreira, M. *et al.* (1998), 'Effects of CLA supplementation during resistance training on body composition and strength', *J. Strength Cond. Res.*, vol. 11 (4), p. 280.

45. Lowery, L. M. *et al.* (1998), 'Conjugated linoleic acid enhances muscle size and strength gains in novice bodybuilders', *Med. Sci. Sports Exerc.*, vol. 30 (5), p. S182.

46. Sebedio, J. L. *et al.* (1999), 'Recent advances in CLA research', *Curr. Opin. Clin. Nutr. Metab. Care*, vol. 2 (6), pp. 499–506.

47. Spriet, L. (1995), 'Caffeine and performance', *Int. J. Sport Nutr.*, vol. 5, pp. S84–S99.

48. Anderson, M. E. *et al.* (2000), 'Improved 2000-meter rowing performance in competitive oarswomen after caffeine ingestion', *Int. J. Sport Nutr. Exerc. Metab.*, vol. 10, pp. 464–75.

Chapter 4

1. Raastad, T. *et al.* (2000), 'Hormonal responses to high- and moderate-intensity strength exercise', *Eur. J. Physiol.*, vol. 82, pp. 121–8.

Chapter 12

1. Fleck, S. J. and Kraemer, W. J. (1997), *Designing Resistance Training Programmes* (Champaign, IL: Human Kinetics).

2. Bompa, T. O. (1996), *Periodisation of Training* (Toronto, Canada: Veritas Publishing).

Chapter 13

1. Bompa, T. O. and Cornacchia, L. J. (1998), *Serious Strength Training* (Champaign, IL: Human Kinetics).

2. Baechle, T. R. and Earle, R. W. (eds) (2000), *Essentials of Strength Training and Conditioning* (Champaign, IL: Human Kinetics).

3. Fleck, S. J. and Kraemer, W. J. (1997), *Designing Resistance Training Programmes* (Champaign, IL: Human Kinetics).

4. Tan, B. (1999), 'Manipulating resistance training program variables to optimise maximum strength in men', *J. Strength Cond. Res.*, vol. 13 (3), pp. 280–304.

5. Hass, C. J. *et al.* (2000), 'Single v. multiple sets in long-term recreational weightlifters', *Med. Sci. Sports & Exerc.*, vol. 32 (I), pp. 235–42.

6. Baechle, T. R. and Groves, B. R. (1998), *Weight training: Steps to Success,* 2nd edn (Champaign, IL: Human Kinetics).

7. Garhammer, J. and McLaughlin, T. (1980), 'Power output as a function of load variation in Olympic and power lifting', *Abstract, J. Biomech.*, vol. 13 (2), p. 198.

8. Hedrick, A. (1995), 'Training for hypertrophy', *Strength Cond.*, vol. 17 (3), pp. 22–9.

9. Westcott, W. L. (1986), 'Four key factors in building a strength program', *Schol. Coach.*, vol. 55, pp. 104–5.

10. Stowers, T. et al. (1983), 'The short-term effects of three different strength-power training methods', *NSCA J.*, vol. 5 (3), pp. 24–7.

Chapter 14

1. Shrier, I. and Gossal, K. (2000), 'Myths and truths of stretching', *Phys. Sportsmed.*, vol. 28.

2. Kokkonen, J. *et al.* (1998), 'Acute muscle stretching inhibits maximal strength performance', *Res. Quarterly Exerc. Sport*, vol. 69 (4), pp. 411–15.

3. Johansson, P. H. *et al.* (1999), 'The effects of pre-exercise stretching on muscle soreness, tenderness and force loss following heavy eccentric exercise', *Scand. J. Med. Sci. Sports*, vol. 9 (4), pp. 219–25.

Chapter 20

1. Herrick, A. R. and Stone, M. H. (1996), 'The effects of periodisation versus progressive resistance exercise on upper and lower body strength in women', *J. Strength Cond. Res.,* vol. 10 (2), pp. 72–6.
2. Bompa, T. O. (1996), *Periodisation of Training* (Toronto, Canada: Veritas Publishing).

Chapter 22

1. American College of Sports Medicine (1995), *Guidelines for Exercise Testing and Prescription,* 4th edn (Baltimore: Williams and Wilkins).
2. Phillips, S. M. (1996), 'Effect of training duration on substrate turnover and oxidation during exercise', *J. Appl. Physiol.,* vol. 81 (5), pp. 2182–91.
3. Smith, J. and McNaughton, L. (1993), 'The effects of intensity of exercise and excess post-exercise oxygen consumption and energy expenditure in moderately trained men and women', *Eur. J. Appl. Physiol.,* vol. 67, pp. 420–5.

4. Kraemer, W. J. *et al.* (1995), 'Compatibility of high-intensity strength and endurance training on hormonal and skeletal muscle adaptations', *J. Appl. Physiol.,* vol. 78 (3), pp. 976–89.
5. 'Weights or cardio first', *Int. J Sports Med.,* vol. 21, pp. 275–80.
6. Osterberg, K. L. and Melby, C. L. (2000), 'Effect of acute resistance exercise on post-exercise oxygen consumption and resting metabolic rate in young women', *Int. J. Sport Nutr. Exerc. Metab.,* vol. 10 (1), pp. 71–81.

Chapter 23

1. Williams, M. H. (1992), *Nutrition for Fitness and Sport* (Dubuque, IO: William C. Brown).
2. Gatorade Sports Science Exchange Roundtable (1998), 'Methods and strategies for weight loss in athletes', *Sports Science Exchange,* vol. 9 (1), pp. 1–5.
3. Friedl, K. E. et al. (1994), 'Lower limit of body fat in healthy active men', *J. Appl. Physiol.,* vol. 77, pp. 933–40.
4. Strauss, R. H. et al. (1993), 'Decreased testosterone and libido with severe weight loss', *Phys. Sportsmed.,* vol. 21 (12), pp. 64–71.

FURTHER READING

Baechle, T. R. and Earle, R. W. (eds) (2000), *Essentials of Strength Training and Conditioning* (Champaign, IL: Human Kinetics).

Baechle, T. R. and Groves, B. R. (1998), *Weight Training: Steps to Success,* 2nd edn (Champaign, IL: Human Kinetics).

Bean, A. (2003), *The Complete Guide to Sports Nutrition,* 4th edn (London: A & C Black).

Bean, A. (2003), *Fitness on a Plate* (London: A & C Black).

Bompa, T. O. and Cornacchia, L. J. (1998), *Serious Strength Training* (Champaign, IL: Human Kinetics).

Fleck, S. J. and Kraemer, W. J. (1997), *Designing Resistance Training Programmes* (Champaign, IL: Human Kinetics).

King, I. and Schuler, L. (2003), *Men's Health: The Book of Muscle* (Rodale).

McArdle, W. D., Katch, F. I. and Katch, V. L. (1986), *Exercise Physiology* (Led & Febiger).

Wilmore, J. H. and Costill, D. L. (1994), *Physiology of Sport and Exercise* (Champaign, IL: Human Kinetics).

GLOSSARY

Actin A muscle protein that acts with myosin to produce muscular activity.

Aerobic In the presence of oxygen.

Agonist (prime mover) A muscle that is primarily responsible for bringing about a movement.

Alpha-linolenic acid An essential fatty acid, belonging to the omega-3 series.

Anabolic The building of body tissue.

Anaerobic In the absence of oxygen.

Antagonist The muscle that acts in opposition to the agonist, opposing the movement.

Atrophy The gradual wasting of a muscle.

Calorie A unit of energy measurement, defined as the amount of heat required to increase the temperature of 1 g of water by 1°C. The common unit used in food labelling is known as a kilocalorie (kcal) and has the value of 1000 calories.

Cardiovascular exercise ('cardio') Exercise that improves the efficiency of the cardiovascular (heart, blood and blood vessels) system.

Catabolic The breaking down of body tissue.

Compound, or multi-joint, exercise Involves one or more large muscle groups and works across two or more main joints.

Concentric The shortening of a muscle during contraction.

Descending (drop) sets A training method that involves performing repetitions to muscle failure followed immediately by further repetitions using a lighter weight until muscle failure is reached again.

Eccentric The lengthening of a muscle under controlled tension.

Eccentric (negative) training Training that involves eccentric action.

Endurance The ability to resist fatigue.

Fast-twitch fibre A type of muscle fibre with a low aerobic capacity and high anaerobic capacity; best suited to speed and power activities.

Forced, or assisted rep, training A method of training that allows you to train past the point of muscular failure; a spotter provides assistance for the last one or two repetitions of a set.

Hypertrophy An increase in muscle size due to increased cell size.

Interval training Repeated brief high-intensity work interspersed with short periods of recovery.

Isolation, or single-joint, exercise Involves smaller groups of muscles and only one main joint.

Isometric A contraction in which tension develops but there is no change in muscle length.

Ligament A strong band of fibrous tissue that connects bones to other bones.

Linoleic acid An essential fatty acid, belonging to the omega-6 series.

Macrocycle A period of training including several mesocycles, usually one season in duration.

Mesocycle A period of training usually two to six weeks long.

Microcycle Period of training, usually one week.

Motor unit The motor nerve and the group of muscles it innervates.

Muscle fibre An individual muscle cell.

Muscle spindles A sensory receptor in the muscle that senses how much the muscle is stretched.

Muscular failure An inability of the muscle to complete another repetition.

Myosin A muscle protein that acts together with actin to produce muscular contraction.

One-repetition maximum The maximum weight that can be lifted for one repetition.

Overload A training load that challenges the body's current level of fitness (e.g. strength) and has the scope to bring about improvements in fitness (e.g. strength).

Periodisation (training cycles) A process of structuring training into periods.

Power The ability to produce both force and speed.

Pre-exhaustion training A method of training that involves performing an isolation exercise prior to the compound exercise to pre-exhaust the target muscle.

Prime mover (agonist) A muscle that is primarily responsible for bringing about a movement.

Progression A gradual increase of workload over a period of time.

Rating of perceived exertion A subjective assessment of how hard you are working.

Repetition One complete movement from the starting position to a position of maximum contraction and back to the starting position.

Set A group of repetitions.

Slow-twitch muscle A type of muscle fibre with a high aerobic capacity, low anaerobic capacity; best suited to endurance activities.

Strength The ability of a muscle to produce force.

Supersets Two or more sets of different exercises performed consecutively with no rest period.

Synergist A muscle that assists the agonists (prime movers) in bringing about a movement.

Tendons Bundles of collagen fibres that connect muscle to bone.

Toning A non-technical term that refers to a relative increase in strength, producing a firmer appearance and feel in the relaxed state.

Training intensity The quantitative element of training such as speed, strength or power.

Training volume The number of sets multiplied by the number of repetitions.

VO2max (or maximum aerobic capacity) The maximum capacity for oxygen consumption by the body during maximal exertion.

INDEX